BUILDING
HEALTHY HUMANS

"This will be the book that I will give to any of my friends that are thinking about getting pregnant or have just become pregnant so they can educate themselves and have the pregnancy and birth that they want the **first time around.**"

-Casey (A Modern Mom)

BUILDING HEALTHY HUMANS

YOUR GUIDE TO A BALANCED AND BEAUTIFUL PREGNANCY FOR A HAPPY HEALTHY BABY

DOCTOR PIA MARTIN

Published by Best Seller Publishing®, Pasadena, CA
Best Seller Publishing® is a registered trademark
Printed in the United States of America.
ISBN 978-1-946978-23-3

Medical Disclaimer:

This book contains advice and information relating to health care. It is not intended to replace medical advice and should be used to supplement rather than replace regular by your doctor. It is recommended that you seek you physician's advice before embarking on any medical program or treatment. All efforts have been made to assure the accuracy of the information contained in this book as of the date of publication. The publisher and the author disclaim liability for any medical outcomes that occur as a result of applying the methods suggested in this book.

This publication is designed to provide accurate and authoritative information with regard to the subject matter covered. It is sold with the understanding that the publisher is not engaged in rendering legal, accounting, or other professional advice. If legal advice or other expert assistance is required, the services of a competent professional should be sought. The opinions expressed by the authors in this book are not endorsed by Best Seller Publishing® and are the sole responsibility of the author rendering the opinion.

Most Best Seller Publishing® titles are available at special quantity discounts for bulk purchases for sales promotions, premiums, fundraising, and educational use. Special versions or book excerpts can also be created to fit specific needs.

For more information, please write:
Best Seller Publishing®
1346 Walnut Street, #205
Pasadena, CA 91106
or call 1(626) 765 9750
Toll Free: 1(844) 850-3500
Visit us online at: www.BestSellerPublishing.org

DEDICATION

I would like to dedicate this book to the fearless and compassionate moms that have shared their very own building a healthy human journey with me.

I have learned so much from all of you and yes it's true every pregnancy is different and unique!!

I would especially like to thank Rachael Adams Gonzales for her faith, trust and belief in the birth process and the power of innate intelligence. She embodies all that it means to be a Modern Mom. A huge thank you "RAG" because if you had not come into my life I would not have had the courage to write this book.

Thank you to Dr. Scott Vrzal for helping me grow as a Doctor and for giving me the confidence to share my message with a larger audience.

The biggest thank you goes to the love of my life. His support, his continued belief in me and his unwavering love has changed my life.

I love you beyond words and this book is your baby too!

SAGE ADVICE FROM SISTERS

My advice is to get to know yourself really well & trust in your wild nature completely. Be gentle with yourself, this is a transition; allow yourself to do things & live in a new & different way. And, ASK for help. Just do it. You're not meant to go at this alone!!!
– Erin

Relax your mind and body. Listen to it, love it, and love the life inside you. Take care of your body and know that what is to come brings HUGE rewards. Don't be scared of the pain, embrace it and soon you will have a beautiful being in your arms that erases all of the hardship and pain before it. **– Alicia**

Trust your instincts; listen to your gut feelings. **– Diana**

Whether it's the delivery or after, things don't always go the way you planned.... and that's ok. Discovering the art of "rolling with it" will become one of your many superpowers. Never forget that there is no one else better than you to give your baby the love, comfort and support he/she needs, whether you are a first timer or veteran.
– Bonnie

It doesn't matter how the baby arrives, how quickly they feed, walk or talk. No one lines up 18 year olds and says - "ooh, I bet you were an early walker." **– Tricia**

Enjoy each moment of your baby's life. Don't always be wishing for when he or she can walk or talk. The time flies by quickly and your child will be grown before you know it. Although there will be many challenges, treasure each day. **– Carolyn**

 The trust because everyone will have something to tell you about how to do this & inside you, you already know the way. **– Erin**

FOREWORD

Written By

A MODERN MOM

My name is Casey and I am the proud mom of two kids. A boy who is a toddler and a little baby girl called Izzy, who is just 4 weeks old.

This is the story so far of how my husband and I created our family.

We wanted to be able use the resources of our modern technological world, however we also wanted to make decisions that were rooted in what is natural and made good sense to us. We wanted balance.

For my first pregnancy, I was so focused on becoming pregnant that I literally forgot about the decisions I would have to make regarding the pregnancy, labor, and delivery.

Once I was pregnant I was excited, however I was also a little fearful some of time. I had lots of questions and was searching for answers that my doctor wasn't providing.

My pregnancy became an anxious struggle as I continued to spend time asking questions, doing research and still not getting sufficient answers.

I was fighting for the birth that I wanted with doctors who appeared to be pushing their own agendas. It was frustrating.

When I decided to get pregnant for the second time, I knew I wanted to do things differently. My new OBGYN recommended that I should consider working with Dr. Pia Martin.

Soon after that conversation I began working with Dr. Pia.

Together we developed a plan that was unique to me that would allow my mind and body to be prepared for a healthy pregnancy.

We worked together for my entire pregnancy. She was the second most important partner (after my husband!) in the process of Building a Healthy Human.

Dr. Pia supported and encouraged me and I was able to have the balanced and beautiful pregnancy I wanted. I was more confident and less anxious and worried, which led to the labor and delivery I desired.

I have grown a lot as a person while working with Dr. Pia, which has helped not only with my pregnancy but it also helped me become a better mother to my first child, and a better person in general. THANK YOU DR. PIA!

I only wish that I had a copy of this book (and Dr. Pia!) prior to my first pregnancy.

This will be the book that I will give to any of my friends that are thinking about getting pregnant or have just become pregnant so they can educate themselves and have the pregnancy and birth that they want the **first time around**.

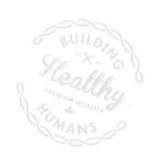

ACKNOWLEDEMENTS

I envision a world where expecting moms and dads value self-care as a priority so they provide their future children with the best start in life.

Every mom wants to have a beautiful and balanced pregnancy and a happy healthy child and to do that it is essential that they provide the building blocks of good nutrition, exercise and emotional stability for themselves first!!

**"You can't give to another what
you do not have yourself"**

A special thanks to everyone who helped and supported me through this journey. Without you, these thoughts and ideas would still be inside my head instead of out in the world supporting others.

To Rob Kosberg and the team at BSP for making the book a reality instead of just a dream.

To Barbie Ray of Barbie Ray Designs, a soon to be new mom, for her beautiful front cover.

To my Editor Stacy code-name Gramma Gal for making my words readable and for her valuable insights and suggestions.

To Dr. Jay Warren for his continued support and for helping me spread the word through his Podcast "Healthy Births Happy Babies."

To Care Messier for her vision and her dreams.

To Dawn Dickerson for her unwavering trust in me.

To Courtney Holst for the internal graphics and the Building Healthy Humans Logo

INTRODUCTION

> We are the only species of mammal that doubts our
> ability to give birth. It is profitable to scare women about
> birth. But let's stop it. I tell women that your body is not
> a lemon.

> —Ina May Gaskin

Why I Decided to Write This Book

I decided to write this book because I envision a world where expecting moms and dads value self-care as a priority so they provide their future children with the best start in life.

Every mom wants to have a beautiful and balanced pregnancy and a happy, healthy child, and to do that it is essential that they provide the building blocks of good nutrition, exercise, and emotional stability for themselves first!

You can't give to another what you do not have yourself!

The real reason I wrote this book is because it is my calling. Some of you might think I am crazy for saying that, but I have tried to ignore it, and the universe was not having it.

Today I am a Doctor of Chiropractic, Certified Clinical Nutritionist and Certified Wellness Coach with a clinical wellness practice in

San Diego specializing in care for pre-pregnant and pregnant moms and babies.

My story started a long time ago; however, my true path became clearer to me only about five years ago.

The real shift started when one of my new mom patients invited me to a Red Tent event. A Red Tent event is where communities around the world hold gatherings as a special place for mothers to share their birth stories, celebrate birth experiences, and heal from traumatic ones. This particular Red Tent is held once a year at The Nizhoni Institute of Midwifery. The Nizhoni Institute is an accredited three-year school that prepares those that have a passion to assist parents and families throughout the birth process with the opportunity to become a licensed midwife.

At this Red Tent event the women who were asked to share their birth stories, were also asked to invite the practitioners who had helped support them through the process of birth and beyond. As you can imagine I was honored; however, it was my very first experience at a natural birth community event.

During the event a doula and HypnoBirthing practitioner and obvious influencer in the community approached me and said we should meet and talk about how I should consider seeing more moms and babies as patients.

"OK," I said nervously. She obviously saw something in me I was not aware of yet! Up to this point in my career as a wellness doctor my exposure to and training with babies and pregnant moms was limited.

I was also suffering from a failed practice partnership, deciding what would be next and working out of my home. I was seriously questioning whether healthcare was the right field for me.

Fast-forward two years and the same mom that invited me to my first red tent event was now pregnant with baby number two.

During her pregnancy she had had some challenges with lower abdominal pain. I asked her to check in with her OBGYN. They found nothing amiss; however, the nagging pain persisted.

At about five and half months pregnant she ended up in the hospital with a fever and an infection. It was a tough time for her and her family. The pain persisted, and I encouraged her after a visit to the hospital to discuss this with the medical staff. They found nothing to support the mom's concerns.

She was sent home and told to rest for the remainder of her pregnancy.

Then my phone rang. "Can you please come to the house and treat me, as I am still in pain?"

I said, yes, I would come; however, inside myself I was not sure what I would do.

As she lay on my table in pain I felt a deep sense of calm come over me, and I began to treat her. When she got up off the table, she said, "This is the best I have felt in weeks."

As I arrived home the phone rang again. Mom had just delivered a baby girl.

It was an OMG moment for me! Mom was only six months pregnant! I was more than a little weak in the knees, and tears were running down my face.

Here is the good news. Baby was breathing on her own and in one of the best NICU centers in the nation and getting great care. Mom was OK but very fragile and would need surgery. They had found that mom had a cyst in her abdomen and if she had not gone into labor and given birth when she did, the cyst would have burst. Mom and baby were lucky to be alive. The care she had received from me had allowed her body to relax enough so she could go into labor. OMG!

As you can imagine, this could have gone the other way, and you would not be reading this book. The experiences with this mom were defining moments for me.

My childhood and relationship with my mother also influenced me. I was thirteen years old when she left my younger siblings and me. When I last saw my mother, a few years ago, she looked like a loaf of bread. She was as wide as she was tall and had a few other characteristics that were not indicative of a healthy lifestyle. She subsequently moved to a nursing home, where she broke her hip trying to sneak an extra serving of ice cream without the nurses knowing. She was a carb and sugar junkie!

Obviously my relationship with my mother was not what I would have wanted. I had no relationship with her for many, many years. However, without her in my life I probably never would have accomplished the things I have accomplished so far. A friend of our family who is very wise says, **"If not that then, not this now."**

It is because of her that I began my journey as a wellness doctor, and it is because of her that I became curious about epigenetics and how we eat, drink, think, and move affects our genetic expression.

But enough about me. This book is supposed to be about you and your unborn baby. I know you are super excited about being a new parent. I also know that you are overwhelmed with all the things you hear and read about: what you should and should not eat and drink and what is best for you and your baby. It seems like everyone is an expert. I know those of you who are first-time parents have some fears regarding the unknown. You have no idea how you are supposed to feel, and frankly, everyone's journey is different and every pregnancy is different.

It is my personal goal to provide a simple, straightforward guide to good nutrition for moms and dads . . . . Right, dads. Dads, it is important for you to be part of the process too . . . Moms need your support.

Everyone is unique and everyone brings their whole self to the pregnancy party, and what is right for one mom is not necessarily right for another.

Sure there are generalities like don't smoke and don't eat sushi and so on. However, I want you to tap into the idea of listening to your body and your baby with mindfulness.

The aim of this book is for you as an individual who brings her whole self to this wonderful journey, to leave with a better understanding of how to tap into motherhood with an understanding that what you do and think is all part of building a healthy human.

This book is my purpose, my passion, and it is written for all those families out there who are searching for ways to improve their health.

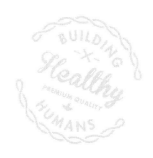

This book is written for pregnant moms and soon-to-be-pregnant moms who

- are curious and want to have a beautiful and balanced pregnancy.
- want to live a health-inspired conscious life that is real and in some cases aspirational yet tailored to their unique concerns and needs.
- were raised using the Internet to answer questions and do research and all too often find the information confusing, and are left feeling stressed and not knowing quite what to do.
- know that the quest for the perfect pregnancy can dominate their every waking thought and action and can ultimately cause major stress, which is counterintuitive to what they desire, which is a happy, healthy baby.
- are somewhere off of perfectionism and more about realism and balance.
- want to feel like their needs and desires for themselves and their new family are considered, and by the way, they do own a yoga mat and make an effort to practice, and they snort a little when they laugh.

"The Doctor of the future will give no medicine but will interest her/his patients in the care of the human frame, in diet and in the cause and prevention of disease"

- Thomas Edison

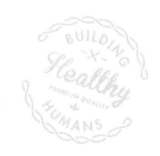

HOW TO USE THIS BOOK

We created this to be a small book, a book that you could tuck into your purse and access when you have a question and need the answer right away.

If you are thinking about becoming pregnant we suggest you start at the beginning, and we hope you agree with us about getting in great shape before you do conceive.

If you are already pregnant, congratulations! You can go to the contents page and easily see the information that applies to you, or read the whole book through to make sure you aren't missing out on anything.

For support and ongoing updates please visit www.drpia.com.

The basic principles you are about to learn apply to all of us who want a more balanced quality of life. Thank you for reading and thank you for sharing and passing the information on to others.

Let's get started!

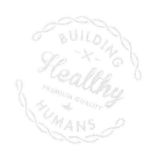

CONTENTS PAGE FOR BUILDING HEALTHY HUMANS

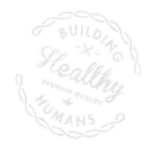

Chapter 1
THE IMPORTANCE OF GOOD NUTRITION

Good beginnings make a positive difference in the world, so it is worth our while to provide the best possible care for mothers and babies throughout this extraordinarily influential part of life.

- Ina May Gaskin

Before I start, know I may say or share things that might be a little different or that you might not agree with 100 percent.

What I want to do is awaken your curiosity and help you really tap in and start questioning what is right for both you and your child.

Here is the good news: You might not have had the best diet growing up and you might have inherited genetics and copied behaviors that are not optimal. However, you can start now by making a conscious effort to improve your life and the lives of your kids going forward.

I mentioned in the introduction that my childhood was not the fairy tale that we all hope for ourselves. That led to my emotional burnout at around twenty years old. I was skinny, sad, and clearly not thriving. I knew deep inside that I needed to make changes. A chance meeting at a coffee shop led me to my first yoga class. One class led to another and another, and soon I was there every morning. I know you may have heard this type of story before; however, this was almost forty years ago when yoga was considered a little underground and maybe even a little cultish.

As I practiced each morning, I started to notice how what I ate affected my physical and meditative practice, so I began to make small changes. Certain foods and drinks would cause my body to feel bloated and stiff, where as other foods and drinks would make me feel limber and light. I experimented a lot back then with different types of diets. I tried a vegan diet, a macrobiotic diet, and many more, and eventually found the clean eating plan that worked for me. That plan is a plant-based paleo diet. http://www.drpia.com. Check out my Plant based Paleo Diet Plan on page 157.

Fast-forward a year or so after I began my daily practice, and I was on my way to India to continue my learning. I was fortunate to spend a year in India with B. K. S. Iyengar, the father of modern yoga and the man who along with Pattabhi Jois brought yoga to the United States. This journey has had a profound effect on the healing of my mind body and spirit. This experience changed my life, and I am forever grateful that is has been part of my journey.

This experience was also the start of the idea and realization that I had actually healed myself without drugs or therapy and that perhaps a career in wellness was my calling. This was a BIG LIGHTBULB moment.

I now have a doctorate in chiropractic, a bachelor's in wellness, and a bachelor's in anatomy. I am also a certified clinical nutritionist, wellness coach and have a thriving clinical wellness practice in Carmel Valley, California, devoted to helping families become the healthiest family they know: http://www.drpia.com.

Generational Health: Dr. Pottenger's Cats

While I was in school studying to become a doctor, I came across a research paper that described an adrenal experiment written by Dr. Price Pottenger, using cats. Dr. Pottenger was an MD who specialized in endocrinology. He conducted various well-documented experiments between 1932 and 1942 that emphasized the importance of a balanced and healthy whole food diet:

> Dr. Pottenger was dedicated to the prevention of chronic illness. In his classic feeding experiments, more than nine hundred cats were studied over ten years. Dr. Pottenger found that only diets containing 100 percent raw milk and raw meat produced optimal health. The consumption of cooked meat and heat-processed milk resulted in physical deterioration, which increased with each generation. https://price-pottenger.org

Dr. Pottenger's research fascinated me and made so much sense to me that I knew his research would become the central idea for this book, as the results and conclusions he made can be seen in human generations.

Understanding the impact of what a pregnant mom eats, drinks, and thinks has on their baby and those of future generations are critical to the overall long-term health of our entire society. A balanced and beautiful pregnancy suggests that we have to make changes in what we eat, drink, and think if we want to have healthy, happy babies.

Here is the short version of one of Dr. Pottenger's landmark experiments:

In this particular experiment he had three groups of cats:

The first group of cats was given food that is found in nature: meat, raw milk, and cod liver oil.

The second group of cats was given some foods that were found in nature with one variant, a food that was processed.

They were given the same raw food and meat. However, Dr. Pottenger gave these cats pasteurized milk—milk that was heated and processed—in place of the raw milk.

The third group of cats was given some of the same foods as the other two groups of cats, with two variants.

They were given the same raw food and meat, but Dr. Pottenger gave these cats **condensed milk**—milk that had been highly processed and also contained a lot of added sugars.

He used cats because they bred quickly and he would be able to document the changes he observed in the cats within a very short time frame.

Dr. Pottenger then documented the changes he observed over a three- generation time span. Any guesses as to the outcome of the groups of cats after three generations?

The **first** group of cats flourished on their diet of natural unprocessed foods, and produced healthy offspring. Their coats were shiny and they had strong teeth and gums. They were playful and interacted well with each other.

The **second** group of cats not so much. He noticed that the first group of kittens born to these mama cats had fur that lacked luster; they had decreased energy, personality changes, and obvious signs of tooth and gum decay. Some also became infested with vermin and parasites. The one small change to processed milk had a significant impact on the health and well-being of the cats.

The **third** and last group of cats on the diet of heat-processed milk with sugar added had all kinds of challenges. By the time the third generation of kittens was born, he noticed remarkable differences. This group of cats had allergies, asthmatic conditions, abscesses, and patchy fur. They also had anxiety disorders, hypothyroidism, and lacked coordination, and if they lived long enough, they were infertile.

WOW! WOW! WOW!

Genes and poor diet were passed on from generation to generation, and the outcome was really grim.

We are seeing these old experiments conducted by Dr. Pottenger being played out today in our own species. Obesity is at an all-time high, antidepressant drugs are the second most prescribed drugs after statins, and more and more women are struggling to become pregnant. We are seeing babies and toddlers with digestive challenges, mood disorders, asthma, allergies, and a host of other immune issues at very early ages.

I know what some of you are thinking. You are thinking you have seen this scenario or something similar in your family or perhaps in a family you know.

I have certainly seen this scenario of how genes and diet affected three generations in my own family:

My mother was a diabetic who broke her hip trying to sneak more ice cream when she was in the nursing home. My brother is a chubby triathlete who lives on carbs; however, due to his level of exercise, he is only pre-diabetic. He is struggling with fatigue, carb cravings, and weight gain. I have a sister who has had trouble with insulin resistance her whole life, and I have to be careful not to let my blood sugar levels get too low.

My brother's daughter is our only representative of the third generation in our family. When she was fourteen years old she started having digestive issues and she struggled with bad acne. She also had challenging PMS and hormonal symptoms. I suggested that she cut out dairy and wheat for thirty days. It was a huge struggle for her to make this lifestyle change, and unfortunately she only lasted two days without her morning hot chocolate and croissant. She was then prescribed hormones (birth control), which helped clear up some of the symptoms. However, this will not address the root cause of her issues. The sad part is that unless she chooses to make changes to her lifestyle, it will for sure catch up with her down the road.

The good news is that if she chooses to make healthier, more balanced diet choices, and exercises regularly, and manages her stress, her body can then heal itself.

Given the Right Stuff, the Body Can Heal Itself

The really good news is that the body can heal itself! Dr. Pottenger conducted another experiment with the cats. He created a fourth group of cats from the second generation of the third group of cats. He began to feed them a raw diet. He wanted to see if the symptoms of the diseased cats would begin to dissipate when they were given raw foods, which were good for them. This group of cats, which had been sickly, began to improve, and eventually they began to thrive.

In my wellness practice most of my patients are seeking help and support on how to **build a healthy human** or to recover from the effects of less-than-optimal genes and poor diet. I am fortunate to see three generations of mostly women in my office all the time: grandma, mom, and baby, or grandma and a mom that is pregnant.

Here is "Mary's" story:

Mary came in to see me when she was twelve weeks pregnant with her second child. She was in tears and full of fear. The birth of her first child had not gone well. It ended with Caesarean Birth, with lots of pain and anxiety during the birth experience. Mary was looking for support and help with her second child so she could have a different experience this time.

We performed an exam on Mary, suggested some dietary changes, and encouraged her to let go of the fear and stress around the birth of her first-born child. A baby that is exposed to chronic stress hormones during pregnancy is pre-programed to be on high alert and can often have issues with anxiety at birth and as a toddler. We want moms to eat well and exercise; however, we also want

6

their pregnancy to be calm and grounded. We want them to have a balanced and beautiful pregnancy.

The story in Mary's own words:

As a newly pregnant mom I was terrified of having the same birthing story I'd had with my son—failed to progress at 9.5 cm with my son being delivered via Caesarean Birth. I saw Dr. Pia throughout my entire [second] pregnancy. She always encouraged me to properly nourish my unborn baby and myself and used a gentle technique to help keep my body in proper alignment for easier birthing. As my pregnancy progressed I decided to attempt a VBAC (vaginal birth after Caesarean Birth). At thirty weeks I had a lot of stress at work and my baby was in the breech position. Dr. Pia used the Webster Technique to encourage baby to turn into the proper position, which was a success! I'm convinced that having my back and hips in the proper alignment not only eased some of the back/hip pain associated with pregnancy, but also contributed to a successful VBAC with my daughter. Thank you, Dr. Pia!

Mary's pregnancy was so different the second time around, and the changes she made to nourish herself and her baby continue to benefit her and her entire family. Mary also encouraged her mom to come in to see me, and here is her story:

I want to say thank you to Dr. Pia Martin for her very gentle adjustments, her gentle nutrition suggestions, and her incredible insight into my health. Although I have been treated by chiropractors for more than twenty years, I have never had the results I have seen with Dr. Pia. I am a solid eighteen pounds lighter and feel so much better. After doing the twenty-one-day cleanse in October 2014, I felt like a different person. My energy levels are up, my joint pain levels are down, my allergies are down, and so many other things. I am now able to recognize (if I pay attention) what my body is telling me about foods—mostly about things I should not be eating.☺ Thank you, thank you, thank you for all you have done for me. Blessings.

This grandmother wants to fix her poor habits, encouraging her daughter to do better than she did, and everyone is focused on giving the new baby the best start. As you can imagine, it is an interesting dynamic. However, it comes from a place of love, and they are in it together seeking a better quality of life for not only the unborn baby but also for themselves.

Here we see the impact of how changes to diet, exercise, and mindfulness transform a family and how outcomes can be improved when you choose to give the body and mind what they need.

It is health that is real wealth and
not pieces of gold and silver.

—Mohandas Gandhi

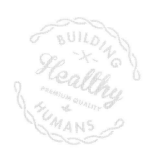

Chapter 2

GETTING STARTED: THINKING ABOUT GETTING PREGNANT

Making the decision to have a child—it is momentous. It is to decide forever to have your heart go walking around outside your body.

—Elizabeth Stone

So you want to have a baby? Well consider yourself fortunate, because by reading this book now and applying what you learn before getting pregnant, you are giving your baby the best chance at health and happiness before they are even conceived.

Your future child's prospects are a delicate balance between your genes and the environment. The two together have an impact on what genes get turned on and expressed and therefore passed on to the next generation, and which genes do not. The most common factors that affect genetic expression are diet, exercise, stress (environmental and emotional), and supplemental nutrition to fill in any gaps.

The rest of this book is designed to provide you with straightforward answers to the many questions that come to mind as you go through your journey of a balanced and beautiful pregnancy for a happy and healthy baby.

Does It Really Matter What a Pregnant Woman Eats?

Yes, it matters! Studies have shown that women who have poor diets actually have a more challenging time in labor, and their babies run a higher risk of infections in their first year of life. Not only that, but they are also more likely to suffer from the long list of pregnancy maladies and increase the likelihood of a Caesarean Birth delivery for their child.

What is also a little discouraging is that you are thrilled with the news that you are going to have a baby and you have received little or no nutritional information from your OBGYN. They are very concerned about the biometrics of pregnancy, like blood pressure, scans, weight gain, etc. However, they provide little or no input into what the quality of the pregnancy should be, and that begins with diet, managing stress, exercise, and supplementing with whole food nutrients.

You have probably heard this statement: "It doesn't matter what I eat, the baby will just take what it needs from my body anyway." It doesn't even sound right, does it? Even if baby takes from mom, do you want a child that survives or one that thrives? When your child is born it might be healthy and intelligent, but how much smarter and healthier could it have been if you had eaten properly? Another thing to consider is, "How can you function as a good parent if you yourself are depleted of nutrients?" Will you have good milk supply, what will the quality of the milk be? Will you heal and bounce back from giving birth? Will you have postpartum depression? Will you be able to handle the stressors that come with having a newborn? I think we have made our point.

THE RIGHT NUTRITION MATTERS! It matters most in baby's first one thousand days, which starts with conception and goes through baby's second birthday. What you feed yourself and your baby will define their wellness blueprint, so MAKE EVERY BITE COUNT!

We are learning more and more about the field of genetics and how environment can affect gene expression. This field is called *epigenetics.*

Epigenetics literally means "above" or "on top of" genetics. It refers to external modifications to DNA that turn genes "on" or "off." These modifications do not change the DNA sequence, but instead, they affect how cells "read" genes.

To understand more about how the factors of epigenetics have influence in the womb, we can look at the results of a famous study conducted at Duke University, which was published in *Molecular and Cellular Biology* (2003). The results of this study on epigenetics reveals to us that we ARE what we eat, breathe, drink, and think, and these factors do affect our genes. Those factors also have an effect on what genes are turned on (expressed) and which ones are not.

Again, yes it matters, and the choices you make now have a lasting effect. Remember the story we told in chapter 1 about Dr. Pottenger and his cat experiments?

Here's another story for you, this time from a mom who was able to change her pregnancy outcome with the right support and a focus on the right nutrition:

Lori's Story

Lori is the type of mom who wanted to make sure she did all the right things during her pregnancy. She followed all of her doctor's orders, had countless tests and scans, and ultimately found herself completely stressed out and diagnosed with gestational diabetes. She then bought her glucose test kit and began to check her levels several times a day in the hopes that she could follow her plan to have a natural birth. The stress mounted, and her OBGYN scheduled her for a Caesarean Birth. This caused Lori to look for another way, someone who would help support her plan to have a natural birth. After searching she found an OBGYN that supported her values, and he agreed to work with her. Her new doctor helped her have her 7.5-pound baby boy naturally.

Lori never gave up on what she wanted for her family.

When Lori decided she was ready to have another child she came to see me. She was looking for nutritional support and wanted to reduce her risk of having gestational diabetes with baby number two. Together we worked on a plan tailored to her unique needs, and she is now twenty weeks pregnant with her second child. She passed her first glucose-screening test with flying colors. Her experience with her second pregnancy is very different than with her first child. She feels supported and listened to and her stress level is much lower than with her first baby. The difference is dramatic. This pregnancy is balanced and beautiful. She is actually able to enjoy the process, and she wants that for all new moms.

How Dad Affects the Genetic Outcome?

You now know that what you eat, think, and do as a mom has an effect on your unborn child, but what about dad? What part does he play?

It goes without saying that having your partner's loving support plays a big part in the health of your child, but dad's role goes further than that.

50 percent of baby's genes come from mom and 50 percent come from dad. Recent research shows that sperm counts have declined 52% in the past 40 years.

With that in mind it just as important that dad have a balanced, healthy diet, keep stress to a minimum, and exercise. Once you have conceived we suggest dads continue the support and play an active role in ensuring the pregnancy is sexy, loving, low stress, and grounded. I am so thrilled to see more dads coming with their partners to their office visits and taking a more active role in co-parenting.

Why You Can't Give to Another What You Don't Have Yourself

We have already briefly discussed why in a perfect and balanced world you would plan your pregnancy. Let's say you did a great job with your first pregnancy and lo and behold you are pregnant with baby number two in less than twelve months. It happens 75 percent of the time. You and your partner get a little careless or are out having too much fun and think, "Well, I am still breastfeeding, so it will be OK. I can't get pregnant anyway." Whoops! Here comes baby number two or three.

I would like you to consider that you might be a little depleted from the first pregnancy and only now starting to feel like you have a good routine in place. I hope you continued to eat well and keep stress at bay; however, I know first-time moms have a tough time. They give 150 percent of themselves to their child and do not take enough time for themselves. I see it all the time in my office. New moms come in frazzled about all kinds of things related to their first child, like the number of poops, the consistency of poops, the number of feeds, how many naps, colic, fussy, crying, birth trauma, and so on.

This behavior causes the stress level of parents to increase and therefore so does the hormone cortisol. Cortisol causes inflammation in the body and over sustained periods of time is damaging to both mom and baby. This is the case even when moms decide not to breastfeed.

Your newborn baby looks to you as its parents to see how you respond to life before he or she responds. If you are anxious and nervous, your baby will be too. Continued and sustained stress increases the cravings for carbs and sugar, which then causes swings in blood sugar, which then causes changes in the microbiome (gut flora), which lays the foundation for a less-than-optimal immune system. Whew!

So as you can see, this cascade of events can lead to a mom and dad that are physically, nutritionally, and emotionally depleted, and most definitely not balanced.

If you want to have more than one child, consider putting the same attention and effort into the first baby as you do for baby number two, three, four, etc. Consider also that your environment affects your newborn child, and make the time to give to yourself too. The idea is to raise a healthy family, which means parents need to take care of themselves. Be a loving and healthy example to your child/children and aim to be the best version of yourself—or better.

Is a Pre-Pregnancy Detox a Good Idea?

As we discussed earlier in the book, in a perfect world you would have planned your pregnancy and you and your partner would have prepared your bodies, your minds, and your spirits by doing a pre-pregnancy detox.

Yes, our P21 program is a good idea!

Here is why:

At one time eating a "healthy diet" and making sure you were taking the right dose of methylfolate was all that was needed. However, in the past decade we've seen a continued escalation in health conditions affecting kids, from allergies (including food and environmental) to asthma, eczema, and autoimmune diseases, and we have also seen a massive rise in the number of kids with autism. Many of these conditions can be traced back to environmental toxin exposure of one or more of the parents of these kids.

These exposures also affect our fertility and genetics that we pass down to our babies at conception.

If you have taken the time to read this far, you know we think providing good building blocks for your soon-to-be-born baby is essential.

We suggest that while you take the bad out, you put the good in. We also suggest that you seek help if you have any health conditions, and work with someone who knows the best way to support you.

If you and your partner live or work in environments where you are exposed to toxic chemicals or metals, then a pre-pregnancy detox is a must! For more see http://www.drpia.com/purification.

You can also go to chapter 3 to learn more on the best foods to eat and why and what foods to avoid. It takes the body time to heal and regenerate. The more less-than-great foods you have been eating, the longer it takes. That makes sense, right?

For a lot of my patients, taking out certain foods is difficult. An example would be gluten, sugar, or soy. If that is the case, go slow. Take out one food group at a time and have fun learning how to prepare healthier foods for you and your family. Our idea of a detox is not radical. Our detox plan is about balance. It's about removing unhealthy food and putting healthy, found-in-nature foods back in. Having said that, some of you might also need some whole food supplement support to fill in the gaps.

TAKING PERSONAL RESPONSIBILITY FOR YOUR WELLBEING IS HARD FOR PEOPLE.

—Bruce Lipton http://www.brucelipton.com

One of our patients, "Vera," decided she wanted to do a hormone reset detox. After she completed her detox, Vera continued to follow a healthy eating and exercise plan. Four months later she was pregnant with her first child. I see these results all the time when moms follow our P21 program.

What if It Is Too Late to Detox?

Life is not always perfect, and sometimes things happen that surprise us. If that surprise is you are already pregnant and all this talk of planning and detoxing is just not going to happen, then you might want to skip the rest of this chapter and go straight to chapter 3.

Chapter 3 is where you will learn how to have a balanced and beautiful pregnancy and a happy, healthy baby, even if you missed the opportunity to detox before getting pregnant.

Foods That Affect Hormones also Affect Fertility

The most common foods that affect fertility are those foods you are sensitive to and that cause a reaction in your body.

You could have a full-blown reaction or it could be something subtle like a rash, a runny nose, or brain fog. You could be sensitive to gluten, soy, dairy, peanuts, and chocolate. Foods you are sensitive to are those foods that create an inflammatory response in the body and therefore affect the gut lining and the microbiome (gut flora). If you continue to consume foods you are sensitive to, over time you could potentially develop an autoimmune-type response, which will typically show up in an endocrine organ.

One example is the thyroid, and the autoimmune diagnosis is called Hashimoto's thyroiditis. A thyroid that is not functioning well has a cascade type effect on the other glands in the endocrine system, and therefore affects the reproductive organs, and therefore affects fertility.

Similarly, a person who is diagnosed with polycystic ovarian syndrome (PCOS) has dysfunctional ovaries, and therefore there is a strong possibility she would have challenges conceiving naturally.

Doing our P21 purification program (http://www.drpia.com/purification) is a good way to eliminate all processed foods and most commonly known allergens. Our program is also a helpful tool because you will learn to recognize if you have a low-grade sensitivity to a certain food. Sensitivities are much harder to detect than an obvious allergy.

Everything you eat is beneficial, neutral, or damaging to your microbiome (gut flora), and therefore foods can have a positive, negative, or neutral effect on your gene expression.

If you are interested in finding out what you might be sensitive to, see your nutritionist or naturopathic doctor and ask them to run an IgG blood test to help identify those foods that impact you. A company called Cyrex Labs has the most comprehensive tests available.

The most common foods that account for 75 percent of all food sensitivity reactions are:

- Wheat and gluten containing foods
- Corn
- Soy
- Processed cow dairy
- Eggs
- Peanuts

We also suggest that you reduce your toxic load as it relates to bath and body products, cleaning products, and air fresheners. These products contain xenoestrogens, which mimic the effects of estrogen, which in turn can affect normal hormonal function.

We have talked about food, environmental toxins, and health challenges and how these factors can have an effect on fertility. Here are a few other things to consider:

- Is your diet low in good-quality protein?
- Are you eating enough high-quality good fats?

- Are you skipping meals and therefore have low blood sugar (hypoglycemic) tendencies? Low sugar causes a spike in cortisol, which has an effect on your hormone levels.
- High blood sugar can also have an impact. If you are overweight and eating too many simple carbohydrates, it is time to re-evaluate your diet.
- Are you under high stress? Take a step back and look at your life and see where you can make some changes. Consider incorporating meditation or some other calming techniques.
- Are you getting enough good minerals in your diet? Increasing your veggies is a good natural way to increase minerals. Adding a green drink also adds big value.

What Are Humans Made Of?

Our bodies are amazing! The body can convert the foods we eat into the basic building blocks for us to grow, repair, digest, and think, and most importantly to provide us with energy.

That being said, some foods are more bioavailable (**take less energy and resources to breakdown into useable form**) than others. Bioavailable foods are those whole foods that are found in nature.

Knowing this, imagine the steps the body must take to convert a food or substance with a lot of chemicals or a ton of preservatives with names you cannot pronounce, into energy. Also imagine how much extra work the liver will have to do to eliminate those toxins from these so-called foods! These foods have little or no nutritional value, yet they require a ton of energy.

Let food be thy medicine and medicine be thy food.

—Hippocrates

So back to our question of what we are made of; the human body is made up of approximately 50 percent water, 30 percent fat, 15 percent protein, 3.5 percent minerals, and 1.5 percent carbs. These numbers differ based on gender, race, etc. However, this gives you a clearer picture of what you might decide to eat if you want to provide the basic building blocks to build a healthy human.

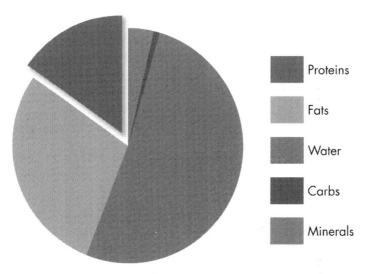

Water

Water is the most abundant building block, and it is important to get enough of it for your body to function efficiently. Staying hydrated is especially important if you are pregnant. Water is needed to form the amniotic fluid and flush toxins that are harmful out of the body to protect your baby.

Note: If you are drinking a lot of water and find yourself peeing a lot, consider adding a little Celtic sea salt to your food. It helps to keep the water in the body by balancing electrolytes. If that does not help, please have your blood glucose checked.

At twenty-eight weeks of pregnancy, your baby is mostly water! So drink plenty of water and add high water content veggies and fruit to your diet.

Fats

Since our bodies and brains need fat, a low-fat diet is a bad idea, especially when you are pregnant and have the desire to have a healthy baby.

Eating the right kinds of fats, like avocados, fish, nuts, and seeds, etc., does not make you fat! Good fats do not cause weight gain. Good fats make you feel more satiated. When you eat foods that are good for you, your body is getting the nutrients it needs.

Good fats are needed to make cholesterol, which is the central building block for cell walls and baby's brain growth and is a precursor for hormones. Good fats also regulate the inflammatory response and help keep your blood sugar stable.

Protein

Protein is used to make the structural components of our bodies. This includes things like tendons, cartilage, muscles, internal organs, skin, hair, and bones. Not all proteins are considered equal. Some are easier to digest than others, and some can cause an allergy or sensitivity reaction. (Think soy or gluten.)

Protein digestion and absorption require good stomach acid. If you have low stomach acid and you have problems with digestion, contact your healthcare practitioner, as you might need to supplement with HCL (hydrochloric acid). Go to chapter 3 for more information on how much protein a pregnant woman needs and what kinds of proteins are good sources.

Minerals

Much of the body is made up of the following key minerals: calcium, phosphorous, and potassium. These minerals are essential for good bone health.

The rest of the body is made up of magnesium, chlorine, iodine, iron, sodium, and sulfur. There are also trace amounts of cobalt, chromium, copper, manganese, selenium, vanadium, zinc, and others. Eating lots of dark green leaves and veggies is where you can ensure you will have a good supply of minerals. Having said that, most pregnant moms will need to supplement to accommodate the needs of their growing baby.

In order to absorb calcium you need good stomach acid, and in order to have good stomach acid you need calcium. As we discussed earlier, if you are having issues digesting protein then you know you are not absorbing calcium. It is possible that you might need to supplement with vitamin D. If vitamin D is low, then it can have an effect on your calcium levels. Have your vitamin D levels checked, and if low get outside for twenty minutes a day and supplement. Optimal levels of vitamin D are 40–80 mg/ml. If your levels remain low you will need to dig a little deeper to see why you are not converting and absorbing vitamin D.

Carbohydrates

Your body needs carbs for energy. However, you should aim to get most of your carbs from vegetables, legumes, low glycemic fruits, and seeds like quinoa. Grains like Basmati rice, buckwheat, amaranth, and farro are also good choices, as most people tolerate them well.

Let's just say that although sugar is a carb, it is not a good carb and causes major endocrine disruption. I know you know, so enough said.

Additional Tests to Consider and Why?

If you have completed a pre-pregnancy purification program and you have been eating, drinking, and thinking well and are still struggling to get pregnant or have some underlying suspicions that you have less than optimal health, it is time to dig a little deeper. Please consider the following additional tests:

1. **Complete Thyroid Panel**

    TSH (thyroid-stimulating hormone) levels are checked regularly; however, TSH tests can often show results that are within the normal medical range. If you are having symptoms such as dry skin, constipation, brittle nails, hair loss, weight gain, being cold all the time, having morning headaches that wear off, and feeling sluggish and/or tired most of the time, you could have an underlying thyroid issue. If this sounds like you, dig a little deeper and ask your physician for further testing.

    We recommend you get checked for T3, RT3, T4, thyroglobulin antibodies, and TPO (thyroid peroxidase). An underperforming thyroid is often an underlying reason for your infertility or miscarriage.

2. **MTHFR Gene Mutation**

    This is a genetic test to see if you can metabolize dietary folate found in plants into the active form of the nutrient. This important gene helps produce methylfolate, the body's most active form of folate. Folate is essential for a number of enzymatic processes and in the developing fetus, and it is essential for the development of the neural tube. The neural tube will later become the baby's brain, spinal cord, and the bones that enclose these structures.

    Folate is a water-soluble B vitamin also knows as vitamin B9 or folic acid.

If you have the MTHFR (methylenetetrahydrofolate reductase) gene mutation (up to 60 percent of us have some challenges converting folic acid into its usable form), you will need to look for the natural form of the vitamin, called **folate**, in your prenatal supplement, not the synthetic form that is called **folic acid**.

3. **Saliva Test**

   A salvia test is useful to check hormone levels that have a direct impact on the ovaries. Those hormones are FSH (follicle-stimulating hormone) and LH (lutenizing hormone). You should also check the stress hormones, which are DHEA (dehydroepiandrosterone), cortisol, and pregnenolone. This test can also be used to test levels of estrogen, progesterone, and testosterone.

4. **Food Sensitivities Test: (IgG [immunoglobulin G], IgA [immunoglobulin A], IgM [immunoglobulin M])**

   This test will tell you what foods you are consuming that could cause an inflammatory response in your body and therefore cause possible changes in your gastrointestinal tract (microbiome).

5. **Vitamin D**

   We suggest that all new moms have the 25-hydroxyvitamin D blood test (abbreviated 25(OH)D). Optimal levels should be mid-range between 40 and 80 ng/ml. Low levels have been linked to possible risks for mothers, like gestational diabetes, preeclampsia, and premature birth. The risks for baby are asthma and behavior challenges.

6. **Vitamin B12**

   This test measures serum vitamin B12 levels. This test is a must if you follow a vegetarian or vegan diet/lifestyle. It is also worthwhile for those who have had stomach problems from poor diet and dysbiosis (disrupted gut flora) and regularly use acid reflux drugs.

What Is Best for My Family and Me?

There is a lot of information out there about what is right and what is not so great surrounding the topic of pregnancy and birth. In fact, you can expect more than your fair share of advice. Random strangers will feel the need to stop you and give you their sage advice. It can all be overwhelming, and this is where you need to tap into what is uniquely you.

You and your partner bring your whole selves to this process of having a balanced and beautiful pregnancy and a happy, healthy baby. It is the sum of your combined experiences, feelings, genes, emotions, etc., that go into making this baby. What is right for one couple might not be right for you.

One of the biggest challenges today is that there is too much information "out there" and not enough information grounded in the natural process of things. Pregnancy and birth is a "natural process" that should be filled with positivity and hope, not worry and fear.

The process of birth can be overwhelming, and before you know it you are concentrating on all the things that could go wrong. Focusing on all the risks, none of the rewards, and you can totally miss the experience. All this stress transfers to your unborn child, which is not good for the baby or you. Trust your body, as it was meant to be able to do this.

Shift your mindset from fear to natural, beautiful, and balanced.

To **prepare your birth plan** for your baby, I encourage you to prepare yourselves with grounding techniques such as meditation, fresh air, walks in nature, yoga, sleep, and deep breathing. Try to stay in the present moment and live it, rather than focus all your energy on worry and fear. Worry and fear live in the future.

If this is baby number two and the first pregnancy did not go as planned, staying in the moment is key because regrets live in the past.

WE WANT YOU TO FEEL GOOD, HEALTHY, SAFE, AND SEXY IN YOUR BODY!

Susan's Story:

Susan was thirty-two weeks pregnant with her first child and she had just learned that her baby was transverse breech. Susan had suspected this, as her belly looked like the head of a hammerhead shark. Susan learned that I was certified in the Webster Technique. The Webster Technique has been shown to be effective in realigning the pelvis and sacrum. Realignment of these areas can relieve distortion and allow baby to move into the proper birthing position. We examined Susan and found that she did indeed have a pelvic misalignment. However, we also learned that Susan was fearful of giving birth and apprehensive about whether or not she would be a good mother. We provided care and gave her a positive mantra to say and think about when she had doubts concerning the upcoming birth.

We saw Susan a week later, and the first words out of her mouth were,

"My baby has turned and is in the proper position, and I am so ready to have this baby."

The adjustment of the pelvis and sacrum plus the mantra and encouragement had provided Susan with some grounding that reduced her worry and fear about the upcoming birth process.

Getting the Best Prenatal Supplement

The key to getting a good supplement is making sure it is bioavailable, which as we said earlier means the body can use it easily. Your prenatal should be sourced from whole foods whenever possible. I like the idea of testing to see whether you can absorb a supplement by using this simple test:

Warm some vinegar to about ninety degrees and drop the supplement into the vinegar and wait fifteen to thirty minutes to see if it dissolves. (The idea is to simulate stomach acid using the vinegar.) If your prenatal supplements do not dissolve, then you know that when you take them, they will go in whole and come out whole at the other end. All that without providing any benefit and using a whole lot of energy.

Check the label for any ingredients that have suspicious sounding binding agents or that have colorings and artificial flavorings. Often a good-quality multivitamin will have all the important ingredients you will need.

From there based on your unique requirements you will most likely need to include additional supplements. Beware of the supermarket brands and read the label. You should be looking for a whole food sourced prenatal tablet or capsule. Go to http://www.drpia.com and click the products link for prenatal options.

Supplements That Fill in the Gaps

The following supplements are intended to fill in the gaps and not to make up for a poor diet. We are assuming you are doing a good job of eating your nutrients. That being said, you are building a healthy human. Many of our foods today are not as nutrient dense as they once were, and even if you are doing a great job of sourcing and eating whole foods, it is highly likely you will need some additional support.

Probiotics

Probiotics provide our digestive system with good bacteria, enabling optimal immune function.

If you have taken antibiotics during your life, then you know that while antibiotics do their job and kill off the bad bugs, they also kill of the good bugs. The gut microbiome can become unbalanced, and that can lead to digestive distress, malabsorption of nutrients, skin issues, allergies, and various other immune problems. Taking a probiotic is about putting the good bugs back into the digestive tract and creating balance.

Good healthy digestion and elimination equals a healthy immune system.

A healthy immune system is good for both mom and baby. The best time to start your probiotic is pre-conception. Probiotics need to be fed inside your gut, so they need good prebiotics. Prebiotics come from indigestible fiber, which is present in many of our denser veggies. Aha! Here is yet another valid reason to eat lots and lots of veggies.

Omega-3 Fatty Acids

These are part of a group called good fats, and they are needed for healthy brain development for baby.

Good fats also reduce inflammation, regulate blood sugar, maintain cardiovascular health, and improve immune function. It is important to look for a good source.

Many of the big chain store products are heat processed and could be rancid, causing increased inflammation instead of actually calming it down. Look for cold-pressed sources from places like Norway. With these products you can be sure the supplement is super clean and does not contain mercury. Krill oil is also a good source of omega-3 fatty acids. If you are vegan or vegetarian you can add flax seed oil, chia seeds, hemp seeds, and black currant oil to your supplement plan. While not an omega-3, evening primrose oil has been used for hundreds of years to address inflammatory conditions and has a rich source of anti-inflammatory omega-6 (GLA).

Vitamin D3

Vitamin D3 is essential for healthy teeth and strong bones. Vitamin D helps with the absorption of calcium and is particularly important during pregnancy. If your levels are low, less than 40 ng/ml (the functional range is 40–80 ng/ml), then you need to supplement to bring the levels up. Getting a safe amount of sunlight every day will also be beneficial. More and more studies show that sunshine is nature's feel-good vitamin.

Magnesium

Magnesium is a co-factor in more than three hundred enzyme systems. It regulates diverse biochemical reactions in the body, including protein synthesis, muscle and nerve function, blood glucose control, and blood pressure regulation. Magnesium is also required for energy production and the removal of toxins from the body. It contributes to the structural development of bones and is required for the synthesis of DNA and RNA, (genetic expression). Magnesium also plays a role in the active transport of calcium and potassium ions across cell membranes. This is a process that is important for healthy bones. Magnesium also helps with muscle relaxation, blood pressure, leg cramps, constipation, and more. Taking magnesium at night before bed can also help with sleep.

B12

B12 is only found in animal protein. If you follow a vegan or vegetarian diet/lifestyle, you will need to supplement with a good source of B12. B12 works with folate to help support proper fetal development and prevent neural tube defects. We also talked about

B12 earlier in this chapter under "What Additional Tests I should consider and why?"

How Does What I Eat, Drink and Think Affect My Baby and Future Generations?

You probably remember the story of Pottenger's cats from chapter 1. If not, I suggest that you go back and read that section now.

Genes and poor diet were passed on from generation to generation, and the outcome after three generations was grim.

We all know families like the group of cats, where the first generation of parents was perhaps baby boomers, the second generation of parents were gen Xs, and now the third generation of parents are called millennials.

Many of the baby boomers (born between 1946 and 1964) were the first group to embrace fast food, low fat, and quick packaged microwaveable meals. They gave birth to the next group (gen Xs, 1965–1984), who hardly ever consumed green veggies or green leaves and who never cooked at home. They then gave birth to the next group (millennials, 1982–2004), who were nutritionally depleted and raised with even more challenges due to the fast pace 24/7 of our world.

The rates of childhood obesity, ADHD, learning disorders, and autism have risen dramatically in the last decade. Is this about better testing, or is it about poor diet and genetic malfunction?

Either way, the good news is that many of the millennial age parents I treat today are looking back and making more conscious decisions. They want things to be different. They want a beautiful and balanced pregnancy and a happy, healthy baby.

They have started a movement to go back to simple, good-for-you food and clean water instead of fast processed food and soda. They are also looking for ways to have less stress and more balance in their lives. Your future child's prospects are a delicate balance between your genes and the environment. The two together have an impact on what genes get turned on, expressed, and passed on to the next generation.

HEALTHY BY CHOICE, NOT HEALTHY BY CHANCE

The importance of a Healthy Gut and Good Digestion

We are hearing a lot these days about *the microbiome*. The microbiome is the delicate balance of good and bad bacteria in the gut. If the gut is upset or you have digestive issues, then chances are good you probably have an imbalance in your gut flora. When the bad guys start to outweigh the good guys, problems start to occur.

That becomes a challenge because 80 percent of our immune system resides in the gut. The gut needs to be healthy, as it digests and absorbs all the vital nutrients needed for building a healthy human, so you can have a healthy, happy baby. A healthy gut also protects and provides you and your unborn child with a healthy immune system.

It was once thought that the mother's womb was a sterile environment. However, new science suggests baby may be exposed to microbes in utero through the placenta.

What we do know and have known for a long time is that as your baby moves through the birth canal, they are exposed to the organisms in your vagina. Hence, this exposure is the beginning of their microbiome and the initial development of their immune system.

There are multiple studies that have proven babies born vaginally have much higher levels of beneficial gut bacteria than those born via Caesarean Birth.

Mother Nature knows how important it is for your child to have a healthy microbiome (balance of bacteria) in the GI tract as soon as possible. The birth process provides your baby with its initial instructions on which to build a healthy immune system. Essentially you transfer your immune system to your child, which is a very good reason to make sure your immune system is in tip-top shape and you have addressed any and all digestive challenges before you and your partner become pregnant.

If you do have to have a Caesarean Birth, then we suggest you follow the instructions below. These instructions come from Maria Dominguez-Bello, who has conducted a wonderful body of research on the topic of birth canal bacteria.

- Insert a piece of gauze into the vagina for one hour before birth.
- Extract before birth, and upon birth wipe the gauze all over the baby, particularly the face and eyes. You will probably want to decline the use of antibiotics, which are often used in baby's eyes at birth.

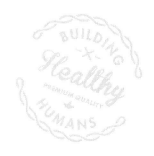

Chapter 3
OMG, WE ARE PREGNANT!

You are pregnant and you are powerful. You are bold
and you are beautiful. Go forward in your boldness,
in your beauty, and in your contentedness. Trust your
body to birth, and know the collective power of women
worldwide will be with you.

—Author unknown

Congratulations! This is an exciting time for both parents. It is also
a time of transition, where there are hormonal, metabolic, and
physical changes going on for mom. If you are first-time parents,
then there are lots of emotions and new experiences. Transitions
are often challenging; however, they lead to incredible growth
and learning.

You have gone from being a woman and a man to being a mother and
father. Dr. Kelly Brogan, http://www.kellybroganmd.com, author of
the book *A Mind of Your Own*, says, "Balancing the woman and the
mother leads to less fear, more love, and freer sense of self. This is
living mindfully in a state of calm alertness."

We started this chapter with quotes about female power and the
naturalness of pregnancy and giving birth. We suggest you create a
mantra for this journey that is positive and powerful and you say it
over and over again until it becomes you.

Ten Best Foods for a Balanced and Beautiful Pregnancy and a Healthy Baby

What you eat is just as important as what you do not eat!

Water

Even though water is a liquid we included it here because of its importance. Many of our nutrient-dense foods contain a lot of water.

Water is one of the basic building blocks of the human body, and when we do not get adequate amounts, our bodies do not work well.

Our bodies are made of 50–60 percent water.

This is especially true for the reproductive organs. Pure water keeps the uterus hydrated and the menstrual cycle running smoothly. Most people do not drink enough water, and many are dehydrated. The guidelines for the amount of water you need are sometimes inadequate and can often fluctuate during pregnancy.

A woman's blood volume increases during pregnancy and at twenty-eight weeks the fetus is made of 84 percent water (not soda or fruit juice.) Aim to drink a gallon of water a day. Start by adding more water over a week to minimize the need to pee every minute. We also suggest that you stop drinking water about two hours before bed so you can have a restful sleep. Be your own best guide. If your lips are dry and your pee is not clear, these are signs you need to drink more water.

Water also helps the bowels work smoothly and is required to replenish the amniotic fluid. **Amniotic fluid** is a clear, slightly yellowish liquid that surrounds the unborn baby (fetus) during pregnancy. It is contained in the **amniotic sac.**

Green Leafy Veggies

Fresh and organic are best. Look to add a variety of the green leafies to your diet to make sure you get adequate vitamins and minerals. A big green salad once a day is a good start.

Green leafy veggies are packed with minerals.

Choose spinach, kale, mustard greens, chard, arugula, etc., and then add in parsley, cilantro, mint, etc. Adding a big handful of spinach to your protein smoothie is another great way to pack in more minerals to your diet. Go to page 159 for our Ultimate Protein Smoothie recipe.

Nuts and Seeds

Nuts and seeds are a good source of protein and excellent as a snack. The best choices are walnuts (omega-3s), cashews, almonds (copper, vitamin E, magnesium), hazelnuts (vitamin E), brazil nuts (selenium), pecans (lots of antioxidants), macadamia (high good fat content), pistachios (rich in copper), and pine nuts (omega-6 and iron). Choose raw organic nuts, and if you like to add some crunch, lightly dry roast in the oven or in a skillet. I really like to eat almonds this way. Toasted nuts are also much easier to digest.

Nuts are among the most nutrient-dense foods nature offers.

We did not add peanuts to the list, as they are legumes and are often associated with mold issues as well as being a common allergen.

Protein

The body is made up of 15 percent protein. The amino acids from protein are the basic building blocks that go into making most of the body's tissues.

A pregnant woman needs 80+ grams of protein a day.

Good sources of foods that are high in protein are lean grass-fed organic meats, organic free-range poultry, wild fatty fish, and organic free-range eggs.

If you are vegetarian or vegan you are going to have to work a lot harder to get adequate protein into your diet while pregnant. Adding a clean protein shake or two to your daily intake is a simple and tasty way to ensure you get the suggested amount. Check protein powders carefully before you buy, and make sure they do not contain added sugar or any suspicious sounding ingredients. We suggest whey protein if you tolerate dairy well, or pea protein if you follow a vegan lifestyle.

In the resources section of the book on page 116, you will find Dr. Pia's Ultimate Protein Shake recipe. Most clean protein powders have between twenty and thirty grams per serving. This is a great way to get a lot of protein, fiber, vitamins, mineral, and phytonutrients.

Colorful Veggies

Colorful veggies are chock full of vitamins, minerals, carbohydrates, and fiber. This is the area where I see a huge opportunity for new moms and most people in general. As a whole we are not eating enough veggies. Aim for five servings a day.

Red Vegetables

Beets

Red peppers

Radishes

Radicchio

Red onions

Rhubarb

*Tomatoes (really a fruit)

Blue and Purple Vegetables

Black olives

Purple asparagus

Purple cabbage

Purple carrots

Eggplant

Purple Belgian endive

White/Tan Vegetables

Cauliflower

Garlic

Ginger

Jerusalem artichokes

Jicama

Kohlrabi

Mushrooms

Onions

Parsnips

Shallots

Turnips

Green Vegetables

Artichokes

Arugula

Asparagus

Broccoli

Broccoli rabe

Brussels sprouts

Chinese cabbage

Green beans

Green cabbage

Celery

Chayote squash

Cucumbers

Leeks

Green onions

Okra

Peas

Green peppers

Snow peas

Sugar snap peas

The nightshade family of vegetables contains lectins. The lectins in nightshades may also be gut irritants in sensitive individuals, setting off a leaky gut response (gas, bloating, constipation, and/or diarrhea).

If you are sensitive to the nightshade veggies, do not consume them, as the body will see them as a toxin. If not, enjoy, as there are many health benefits from most members of the family Solanaceae.

Nightshades:

Tomatoes

White potatoes

Peppers (all kinds)

Goji berries

Eggplant

When healing from an autoimmune disease (especially rheumatoid arthritis or anything else that causes joint pain and inflammation) a thirty-day nightshade elimination diet is definitely worth a shot. After all, it can't really hurt, and you might be surprised at the benefits.

Good Fats

We have been trained for years and years that fat is not good for us and it can cause heart disease and obesity. We have since learned that this is not the case and that all fats are not created equal. The body is made up of approximately 25 percent fat, less for men and slightly more for women. Fat is the primary building block that allows the liver to make cholesterol. Cholesterol is the precursor used to make hormones, the cell walls, and most importantly, the brain.

A low-fat diet during pregnancy is a bad idea, and contrary to popular belief, you will not get fat eating good fats—you will get fat eating too many carbs.

Good fats promote fertility.

Fats provide a lot of energy, almost twice as much as carbohydrates. If you are vegan or vegetarian, good fats are a must, as they will also help stabilize your blood sugar. As we said earlier, good fats support the synthesis of cholesterol, the precursor to better hormone production, and therefore also promote fertility. Trying to conceive? Then we suggest you and your partner increase your good fat intake.

Good fats are avocado, coconut oil, grape seed oil, olive oil, flax seed oil, algae, organic butter or Kerrygold, ghee, egg yolks, lean meats, fatty fish, and nuts.

A word about dairy: We suggest a limited amount of dairy, especially if it is processed cow dairy or if you have sensitivity to the protein casein (the protein found in dairy products). Butter does not have as much casein, and therefore people that are sensitive to cow dairy can tolerate grass-fed butter like Kerrygold. Dairy might not be a problem for everyone; however, if you choose to consume cow dairy please make sure it is organic and whole. Also try goat and sheep dairy options.

Unhealthy fats are modern processed oils, which are industrially manufactured from GMO crops. They are corn oil, soybean oil, safflower oil, canola oil, and cottonseed oil. Also avoid all foods with trans fat.

If has been shown that the placenta protects baby from bad fats to some degree; however, I would not want to put this to the test. You, mom and/or dad, also need to stay healthy.

Olive Oil Fraud

A lot of imported "olive oil" is actually a combination of olive oil and cheaper, refined oil. To protect yourself, opt for olive oil with the California Olive Oil Council (COOC) logo on the bottle.

For olive oils from France look for the AOC logo; from Italy, the DOP logo; and from Spain, the DO seal.

Source: Berkeley file://localhost/Wellness http/::www.berkeleywellness.com:healthy-eating:food-safety:article:beware-food-fraud

Fruits

Fruits and veggies are often talked about as one food group and in the same breath. The fact is, fruits contain different types and different amounts of sugars than veggies.

The type of sugar found in fruit is fructose, and it can lower insulin sensitivity and cause blood sugar swings. This is a problem area as it relates to the glucose tolerance test. We suggest that you choose fruits that are low on the glycemic index: like berries, lemons, limes, pears, pineapples, etc. Aim to eat twice as many veggies as you do fruit.

We like adding lemon or lime to our water to make sure we get extra vitamin C and flavor, and we like adding berries to our protein shake for some fiber and sweetness.

Spices and Flavorings

We have been learning more and more about the healing properties and anti-inflammatory benefits of spices. Find ways to add these nutrient-dense gems to your diet. They include ginger, turmeric, cumin, cinnamon, allspice, mustard seeds, garlic, onions, cilantro, sea salt, and apple cider vinegar, just to name a few.

Try adding spices and flavorings to homemade salad dressings, or make a Thai- or Indian-style curry, or add them to your high protein shake for some added flavor.

Adding ginger to make a tea is a great way to sooth digestion and calm nausea. Ginger neutralizes the acids in the digestive system that causes nausea, cramps, vomiting, and diarrhea. Ginger also reduces inflammation and acts as a natural antihistamine and antifungal.

Whole Grains

Limit your grain intake. If you choose grains, choose whole sprouted grains. We like to use grains as a garnish instead of a whole meal. Make the switch to having more veggies on the plate and fewer grains.

Quinoa has been called an ancient grain and touted for its nutrient benefits. In some circles quinoa is considered a seed. It is high in protein, gluten-free, and high in antioxidants.

Refined carbohydrates promote unstable blood sugar.

- Important: Beware of processed products such as pastas or breads made out of quinoa flour. These products are usually refined and may not contain the health benefits of eating the grain whole. Processed quinoa products can be used occasionally as a substitute for wheat-containing options.

We strongly suggest you eliminate all refined carbohydrates and flour, as these foods promote unstable blood sugar, which is the last thing a soon-to-be pregnant or pregnant mom wants.

Bone Broth

For thousands of years, there have been traditional foods like fermented veggies and cultured dairy that have been touted for their health benefits. But one common healing food that is now being recognized for its incredible health benefits is bone broth. Why is that? Bone broth contains collagen, which is a central building block for a variety of structural tissues, like bones, ligaments, and cartilage. Collagen is also a key component found in skin, hair, and nails, and supports the intestinal lining of the digestive tract.

Chicken soup isn't just good for the soul.

There's a reason chicken soup has been prescribed by doctors and mothers alike when you're feeling under the weather. That's because bone broths are nutrient-dense, easy to digest, rich in flavor, and also boosts healing.

Bone broth or stock was a way our ancestors made use of every part of an animal.

Nutrition researchers Sally Fallon and Kaayla Daniel of the Weston A. Price Foundation http://www.westonpricefoundation.com explain that **bone broths contain minerals in forms that your body can easily absorb. These minerals include calcium, magnesium, phosphorus, silicon, sulfur, and others.**

One of the most valuable components of bone broth is gelatin. Gelatin provides us with building blocks that are needed to form and maintain strong bones, and it supports healthy bone mineral density.

It's recommended to consume eight ounces one to two times daily as a soup or a plain beverage to get all these wonderful bone broth benefits. You can make it yourself, it can be found frozen in health food markets, or it can be found in powdered form and added to your daily shake. Make sure it is organic.

The following is a simple recipe for making your own bone broth at home.

Healing Bone Broth Recipe

1. Place five pounds of rinsed and cleaned chicken bones into a 6-quart slow cooker and cover with water.

2. Add two tablespoons of apple cider vinegar to water prior to cooking. This helps to pull out important nutrients from the bones.

3. Fill stock pot with filtered water. Leave plenty of room for water to boil.

4. Bring to a boil and then reduce heat to simmer for at least six hours. Remove scum as it arises.

5. Cook slow and at low heat. Chicken bones can cook for twenty-four hours. Beef bones can cook for forty-eight hours. A low and slow cook time is necessary in order to fully extract the nutrients in and around the bone.

6. You can also add in vegetables, such as onions, garlic, carrots, and celery, for added nutrient value.

After cooking, the broth will cool and a layer of fat will harden on top. This layer protects the broth beneath. Discard this layer only when you are about to eat the broth.

What Foods to Avoid

My intention in writing this book was to focus largely on the positive aspects of a balanced and beautiful pregnancy for a happy, healthy baby. However, it is important to address the foods you should avoid. We also want to help you understand why you should avoid these foods, as many of them can potentially harm your unborn child.

We challenge you to avoid many of these foods for the rest of your life and the lives of your children. After all, shouldn't you take great care of yourself always?

Junk and Fast Foods

Up to two hundred chemicals have been found in the umbilical cords of some babies. This is a very good reason to avoid a quick stop at a fast food outlet. These foods have little to no nutrients and lead to blood sugar swings that have a big impact on hormonal health and morning sickness.

Sugar is not a nutrient-dense choice for you or your baby.

Sugar and Sugar Substitutes

What you eat, your baby eats. Sugary snacks and foods have no nutritional value and lead to blood sugar swings, which have a huge impact on fetal development. Keeping blood sugar stable will help you avoid nausea, **morning sickness**, problems with **gestational diabetes**, anxiety, cloudiness, irritability, and the jitters.

Trans Fats and Vegetable Oils

We discussed this and olive oil fraud earlier in this chapter under "Good Fats," if you need to review it.

I'd like to add here that it has been shown that the placenta protects baby from bad fats to some degree. However, I would not want to put this to the test. You, the mom and/or the dad, also need to stay healthy and well.

If you eat out ask your server how they cook their food. Most fast type restaurants use processed vegetable oils.

Processed Grains

We often are told that it is OK to have lots of little carb snacks all day long to keep our blood sugar stable. Umm . . . I think if you have been reading this book you know how we feel about this statement. Again, what you eat, your baby eats. Almost all processed grains have added chemicals and sweeteners. If the label says "natural" or "organic" and it comes in a box or a packet, it is processed. Check the ingredients before you consume.

Alcohol, Drugs, and Cigarettes

This is obvious; however, if you need to take drugs or have a health concern, please check in with your OBGYN. It would also be worth your time to consult a wellness practitioner to help you with the root cause resolution for what ails you.

What about a glass of wine? Your body goes through a myriad of hormonal changes during pregnancy, and those hormones affect the entire endocrine system. In fact, the liver is an endocrine organ, so using things metabolized by it during pregnancy (like alcohol and many drugs) puts extra stress on this vital organ.

The liver will metabolize alcohol before it metabolizes toxins.

Soft Drinks

If you can, wean yourself off of soft drinks before pregnancy, and never ever choose to drink them again. If you choose to drink them postpartum, you will have a very difficult time keeping your kids away from them. They see what you and hubby drink and eat, and they will want what you drink and eat. The cycle of poor diet and unhealthy behaviors will keep on perpetuating itself.

What about Coffee and Other Drinks?

There are lots of conflicting opinions on what is safe.

Here is what we know: Caffeine blocks the absorption of iron and raises your cortisol levels, which then impacts the adrenal glands.

There is a lot of discussion out there about coffee. Here's how you need to think about coffee. Coffee oftentimes raises cortisol levels in the body. Cortisol is the stress-handling hormone secreted from the adrenal glands in response to stress.

Due to the hormonal changes taking place during pregnancy, it is vital that the adrenal glands are strong and stress is kept to a minimum. Pregnancy is stressful, and the adrenals need to be strong in order to have the healthy pregnancy you want.

High cortisol has an impact on energy levels, blood sugar levels, and much more. If you do choose to have coffee, we suggest you have only one cup a day and choose to enjoy it with coconut milk, goat milk, full-fat organic milk, or half and half. The fat in the coffee will slow the release of caffeine into the body. We also suggest that you keep an eye on your iron levels.

Other Drinks

We strongly suggest that you avoid sugary drinks like sodas and alcohol. Stick to plain water with a spritz of lemon in it. Protein shakes are also a great idea. For the Ultimate Protein Shake recipe go to page 116.

High Mercury Fish

Avoid tuna, swordfish, and shark, as they are large and accumulate mercury. Mercury is a toxic metal, and it impacts brain function. 'Nuff said.

Raw Seafood

It is best to avoid raw seafood, including raw sushi, due to possible complications from parasites and worms.

Soft Cheeses

Soft cheeses are made with unpasteurized milk that may harbor Listeria bacteria, which can be life-threatening for mom and unborn baby.

Raw Eggs

It is best to avoid raw eggs due to the possibility of Salmonella bacteria. Say no to homemade Caesar dressing, hollandaise sauce, and mayonnaise.

Mixed Bag

- **Deli meats** and hot dogs: They contain a myriad of chemicals and have been known to contain Listeria bacteria.
- **Chinese food:** More often than not it contains MSG. MSG is an excitotoxin and very damaging to the body and more importantly the brain.
- **Soy:** If you choose to eat soy look for fermented organic sources. Soy is pro-estrogenic and can mimic estrogen and upset the hormonal balance of the body. The other concern with soy is that it is highly processed and genetically modified (GMO).
- **Peanuts:** As we talked about earlier, peanuts are a high-risk food and allergen and known to contain mold. Peanuts are not nuts. They are legumes. So can peanuts be healthy? Yes, they can be if you buy high-quality, organic peanuts like Valencia peanuts and you get plenty of omega-3 fats in your diet to offset the high amount of omega-6 fat found in peanuts.

    But here's the problem: 99 percent of the peanut butter and the peanuts people buy in America have hydrogenated oils added, and they're non-organic. That's what adds to the omega-6 count and makes peanut butter unhealthy. Sadly, 99.9 percent of peanut butter out there today is absolute junk. It's not good for you, and it can even cause weight gain and inflammatory reactions in the body.

- **Dairy:** Choose organic sources from grass-fed cows. A special note: The primary protein in cow's milk is **casein,** which is difficult for the body to digest. Pasteurization transforms lactose found in milk into beta-lactose sugar, which causes rapid absorption, spikes blood sugar, and therefore increases insulin. **Remember, cow dairy is highly processed; therefore, choose organic pasture-raised raw sources.**

  The harmful parts of the milk proteins are only present in very small amounts in butter, and they are enzymatically modified during the butter pasteurization process. For this reason, butter can be a good choice as a fat.

- **Herbal tea:** We suggest you consume herbal tea with caution. There is a lot of conflicting data about what herbs are and are not safe for pregnant moms. The other question is the quality of the herbal products that are available. Are you sure of the source?

  Most herbs are contraindicated for pregnant and lactating moms; however, some midwives suggest raspberry leaf tea to help with delivery. I would enjoy fresh herbs like parsley, ginger, and rosemary in my foods in moderation. A special note: Green tea increases the need for folic acid. So if you want to have green tea, make sure you are getting adequate folic acid in its active form: folate.

Understanding Morning Sickness and Reducing the Symptoms

Morning sickness is one of the ways a woman's body protects baby from the toxins in food. Toxins make everyone sick, and women who are pregnant are much more sensitive to toxins, particularly in the first ten to twelve weeks of pregnancy.

The change in your hormones is causing fluctuations in the entire endocrine system, and women that experience other endocrine challenges or a compromised digestive track are often more likely to have problems with morning sickness.

Toxins make everyone sick, and pregnant women are much more sensitive.

Here's another way to think about morning sickness:

You have found out that you are pregnant, so wanting to make sure you have a healthy baby, you suddenly cut out a bunch of foods and drinks from your diet.

If they were foods and drinks you were consuming on a regular basis (an example would be coffee), the body will go through a detox process.

So not only are you dealing with the changes in hormones, but you are also going through a mild to moderate detoxification. If your liver function is very good, then you might have a mild headache and be fine. If your liver is not functioning optimally then you will probably struggle with nausea and fatigue. This mechanism is there to protect baby while your body rids itself of toxins.

The first twelve weeks are very important in early development when cell division is very rapid. By the end of twelve weeks your baby is fully formed.

Since your baby's most critical development has taken place, your chance of miscarriage drops considerably after three months into the pregnancy.

Here is a balanced and mindful way to think about food cravings. We mostly crave foods that are not good for mom and/or baby.

Before indulging, ask yourself the question,

"Does my body want or need this, or is it something else?"

If you are craving things like ice or metals, then that is another story. You should check in with your practitioner because there could be a more serious issue going on.

Here are some other possibilities that could be the root cause of your nausea and morning sickness.

> **Adrenal stress:** If the adrenals are weak, the changes that occur during the early stages of pregnancy can cause morning sickness. We have had good success in treating and supporting the adrenal glands.

> Stressors to the adrenal glands could be physical, emotional, or nutritional. What we mean is too little or too much in either one of these areas.

> **Other hormonal challenges:** The endocrine organs work on a positive and negative feedback system. If you have dysfunction in another endocrine organ, then that could have an impact on morning sickness. Examples would be, PCOS (polycystic ovarian syndrome), blood sugar challenges like hypoglycemia or insulin resistance, uterine fibroids, and a history of PMS. Not enough sleep can cause disruption, so can thyroid challenges and/or liver and gallbladder dysfunction. If you know you have endocrine challenges, our P21 program should be part of your plan.

If you do feel nauseous, try to eat protein and fat first and not simple carbs. Try to eat small meals often and pay attention to triggers. For some people ginger is helpful, as it aids in digestion and neutralizes acids that can cause nausea and vomiting.

Ginger also acts as an anti-histamine and is anti-fungal. Last but not least, the healthier you are going into pregnancy, the less you will experience morning sickness. http://www.drpia.com/purification

In our office we have success reducing morning sickness symptoms by supporting the adrenal glands and adding digestive enzymes and liver support.

How Much Protein Do I Need?

Pregnant women need between 80- 90 grams of protein a day for a healthy pregnancy. Proteins provide the essential amino acids needed to build a healthy human. Not enough protein and the body will take it from muscle, which will deplete muscle mass, too much will put a strain on the kidneys and liver.

The body does not store amino acids, therefore we suggest that you aim for 25 grams per meal and then add a high protein snack like organic raw or dry roasted nuts to hit your daily target.

To help you understand what eighty grams of protein should look like on a daily basis we have included and example.

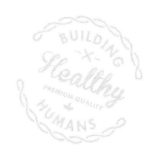

Here is what 80+ grams of protein look like.

PROTEIN TYPE	KITCHEN MEASUREMENTS	GRAMS
Lean Grass Fed Beef	6 ozs	54 grams
Turkey		51.4 grams
Chicken, dark		48.6 grams
Chicken, white		37.8 grams
Fish (Salmon, Halibut, etc)	3 ozs	22 grams
Almonds	1 cup	20 grams
Peas		10 grams
Black Beans		15 grams
Hummus		12 grams
Lentils		18 grams
Oatmeal		11 grams
Quinoa		8 grams
Plain Greek Yogurt		10 grams
Spinach, cooked		5 grams
Broccoli		4 grams
Pumpkin Seeds	1oz	5 grams
Peanut Butter		7 grams
Tempeh		5 grams
Chia Seeds	1 teaspoon	3 grams
Spirulina		2 grams
Egg	One	6.3 grams

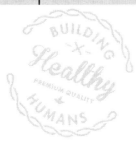

What if I Follow a Vegan or Vegetarian Diet?

Here are some of the pitfalls we see when moms follow a vegan and vegetarian diet. Moms tend to consume:

Too many simple carbs and not enough veggies

Vegetarian and vegan moms also tend to consume too much soy protein, which for some can contribute to thyroid problems. We discussed how the endocrine system is linked and how one gland can affect another. The increase and shift in hormones during pregnancy can affect the thyroid. Soy has also been identified as an allergenic food, and there is lots of speculation as to the genetic modification of this food. So with that being said, stick with organic and fermented sources of soy, like tempeh, miso, and tamari.

Another challenge we see for vegan and veggie moms is keeping up with the amount of suggested protein their growing baby needs. Please check out our protein guide located page 52 to help ensure you are getting a variety of foods in adequate amounts.

We also suggest you make sure to consume plenty of good fats, deep pigmented veggies, nuts, and seeds. Women who typically follow a vegan or vegetarian diet often struggle to keep their blood sugar in a healthy range. Again, saying it twice, if you are a vegan or vegetarian mom, I strongly encourage you to make sure you get plenty of good fat, lots of nutrient dense colorful veggies, and high-quality protein.

What if I Follow a Paleo Diet?

Here are some of the pitfalls we see when moms follow a strict paleo diet: Moms then tend to consume too much meat, and the meat is often from questionable sources. Also the kinds of meats (bacon, pork etc.) consumed can contain nitrates that have been shown to be harmful for baby.

As a soon-to-be new mom you have to be careful about keeping the right balance to ensure you get all the nutrients needed for your growing baby. Again, as with vegan and veggie moms, paleo moms do not consume enough deep-pigmented veggies.

A high protein diet can also be very taxing to the kidneys, and therefore can cause challenges with digestion and constipation.

Personally, I am a pegan, or you might say I follow a plant-based paleo diet (if we have to put a label on our diets). This type of diet works best for me. It makes me feel balanced. It consists of lots of veggies and greens, nuts and seeds, good fats, some low-glycemic fruits like berries and pears, and lean proteins, mostly from wild fish and fowl. If you are interested, there is a simple plant-based paleo diet outline in the back of the book. Remember, this book is about finding your balance and what is right for you.

How Much Weight Gain Is Healthy

Here's what the guidelines for BMI (basal metabolic index) suggest if you fall into what is considered the normal range.

You can calculate BMI yourself: BMI is your weight (in kilograms) over your height squared (in centimeters) http://www.bmi-calculator.net

That range is between 18 and 25. If you are in this range, then the average and healthy weight gain is between twenty to thirty pounds with twenty-five pounds being the average. That being said, it is a myth that you need to eat for two. You probably don't need many more extra calories until you reach the third trimester. What counts is the quality of the calories you consume, not the quantity.

If your BMI is less than 18 you should gain some healthy weight. If your BMI is 25–30 or higher, then you are overweight, and therefore you should gain less weight to avoid pregnancy problems down the road.

If you are overweight and want to get pregnant, I strongly suggest you seek support prior to conception. It will be much better for you and much better for baby.

Keeping My Immune System Strong

The best way to keep your immune system strong for a balanced and beautiful pregnancy is to eat well, exercise, and **keep stress to a minimum:**

- Avoid simple sugars and simple carbs.
- Enjoy lots of greens.
- Get adequate calcium, magnesium, and vitamin D3.
- Take a good probiotic.
- Download the app called "Headspace" and meditate: http://www.headspace.com.

Gut health is critical for managing immune health. Enjoy your pregnancy and celebrate all the things you do each day to nurture yourself and your baby. If this is your first pregnancy try to stay balanced and not stress about every detail. Stress has a huge impact on the immune system and therefore a big impact on the health of your baby.

Stay grounded and stay in the moment. Love yourself and love your baby.

I Am Sooo Tired. Handling Fatigue

Your body is going through a lot of big changes at a fairly rapid pace so you are going to need additional nutrients to support these changes.

First: Make sure you are getting adequate sleep. The body repairs itself during sleep, and that is when the liver does most of its work to rid the body of toxins.

Second: Dehydration could be the cause of your fatigue. Make sure you are getting plenty of fresh water, at minimum 80 oz. per day. As discussed you will need even more in the third trimester.

Third: Toxins could also be a likely culprit. If you are eating poorly and mismanaging your blood sugar, you will feel tired.

If you are getting good sleep, eating well, and are well-hydrated and still feel fatigued, you should check in with your physician to make sure you do not have a hidden infection or are low in a specific nutrient.

Your fatigue could also mean you need more nutrients, especially folate, B12, vitamin D, and B-complex. (A special note about iron: Unless your blood work shows a deficiency, we suggest eating foods rich in iron. Supplemental iron can cause digestive stress and is difficult to absorb.

You should also make sure your prenatal vitamin is high quality.

You can self-test the quality of your prenatal supplements by dropping them into white vinegar that is heated to ninety-nine degrees. If they dissolve in thirty minutes or less, then your body will absorb them. If they do not dissolve completely, then you have just learned that you have expensive pee and it is time to upgrade your prenatal vitamin. For suggestions go to http://www.drpia.com and click the Products button.

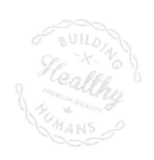

Chapter 4
THE SECOND TRIMESTER: THE HONEYMOON STAGE

If you think taking care of yourself is selfish, change your mind. If you don't, you're simply ducking your responsibilities.

—Ann Richards.

Staying the Course with Good Nutrition

For most women the second trimester is the period of time when they feel good, and some moms even feel really great. You have a baby bump, your hormones feel in balance, your nausea it has subsided, and your energy level is back to normal.

If you had some struggles during your first trimester trying to eat all the nutritious foods we talked about in chapter one and two, then this is the time to make a better effort. It is never too late to do this, and better late than never.

Don't beat yourself up about the past; just start now and look forward and stay grounded in the present moment.

This is also the time that you should have more energy, so it is time to get back on track with a regular exercise routine or sign up for a prenatal yoga class in your area. (This is also a great way to meet other pregnant moms.)

Baby's Bones Are Developing: Why You Need Magnesium, Calcium, and Antioxidants

The second trimester is the time when your baby is developing skin and bones. This is a period of time when there is rapid growth and a need for the minerals that build strong, healthy bones. We talked a bit about the many benefits of magnesium in chapter 3. Remember magnesium also works in conjunction with calcium and phosphorus to build bones.

If you are following a healthy eating plan and you are filling in with whole food supplements you should be getting enough of these important bone-building nutrients.

This is a time when collagen is also important. We talked a bit about collagen in chapter 3, so you already know it is a key building block for many of your baby's structural tissues like cartilage, tendons, and ligaments, as well as healthy skin, nails, and hair. One of the central building blocks for collagen is vitamin C. Fortunately, vitamin C is found in a lot of foods. Adding a squeeze of lime or lemon to your drinking water is an easy and good way to make sure you are getting vitamin C in a natural form.

Ramping Up the Calories a Little

I am a little reluctant to suggest this, as most moms will take me at my word and perhaps over-indulge. As we discussed earlier this is a period of rapid growth for your baby. You will need to up the calories a bit to accommodate this growth spurt.

We suggest making sure you are eating adequate protein and good fats. These are the two areas to focus on to ensure you are getting enough of the right kind of calories. Refer to our protein guide on page 52 for more information.

The other thing to mention here is that you are not actually eating for two. It is key to really listen to your body. If you are in tune and connected with your body you will know what you need.

Why All Calories Are Not Created Equal

The quality of the food you eat is extremely important. The term "calorie" is used a lot, and it is a measure of energy we still see used in conjunction with weight loss programs and the like.

For example, if you gained one pound or lost one pound without changing anything, you would have added or taken away 3,500 calories, respectively.

That being said, what you want is to consume food that is nutrient dense so you obtain the maximum benefits for your unborn baby and yourself.

The other interesting thing is, when you eat nutrient-dense food you feel more satisfied and more energized. When you eat empty calories, your body does not get the nutrients it needs, and therefore you feel hungry.

Your body thinks it is starving because your body and brain are malnourished.

Staying Hydrated: Water, Water, and More Water

Staying hydrated during pregnancy is very important. As discussed earlier water is a key building block for a healthy baby, and it is especially important during the formation of the amniotic fluid early in the first trimester.

Again, if you are drinking plenty of water but it seems to be going right through you, add a pinch of sea salt or Himalayan salt (for electrolytes) to your water. You might also need other additional electrolytes, and if so please talk to your health practitioner about what is best for you.

We also suggest that you don't drink water out of plastic bottles, that the water is filtered and best consumed at room temperature.

Some of the negative symptoms associated with pregnancy such as muscle cramps, headaches, constipation, fatigue, etc., are often signs of dehydration and can be easily cured by drinking enough clean filtered water. If you hate drinking water, add some lemon, cucumber, or pineapple to give it a little flavor.

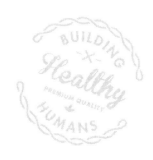

Chapter 5
PREPARING FOR BIRTH

The third trimester is a time when your unborn child has completed the development of their major structures with some fine-tuning still to be done. This is the time when your child grows rapidly and prepares to live and thrive outside the womb.

All of a sudden it will seem like you are carrying this huge ball in front of your body that you need to accommodate. Your center of gravity changes and the extra weight along with the change in your silhouette can cause uncomfortable back and pelvic pain.

Keeping up with your prenatal yoga, exercise of your choice, and healthy food choices are as important as ever. The added stress of the weight gain and additional fluid volume can definitely take a toll on your body.

If you have not done so already you might want to consider adding prenatal chiropractic care, acupuncture, or prenatal massage to your pregnancy care plan.

This is also a time of great joy as you prepare to celebrate with friends and family by planning a baby shower or a ceremonial blessing. It is also a time to finalize the plan you and your partner would like for the birth of your beautiful baby.

For a balanced and beautiful birth, I highly recommend that couples take a HypnoBirthing class: http://www.birtheducationcenter.com. HypnoBirthing classes help parents prepare emotionally and spiritually (whatever that means for you) for the magical experience of birth and what it means to bring a child into the world. This is a great class for dads because it prepares them for the reality of their role up to, during, and post birth of your baby.

HypnoBirthing teaches you how to go into the moment of calm during the birth process, which has huge benefits. That calm place of being reduces stress and allows the body to stimulate oxytocin. Oxytocin is the hormone that allows "relaxin" to do its work on the muscles and ligaments for an easier birth process.

Avoiding Late Pregnancy Problems

We hope you have been eating a clean healthy diet, exercising regularly, and keeping stress to a minimum and therefore do not have any late pregnancy problems. However, if you do, we wanted to provide you with some suggestions and support.

About Gestational Diabetes

I decided to write this section because I kept seeing that more and more new moms are having blood sugar problems during pregnancy. I also found that moms were having a challenge finding information that was straightforward, made sense, and provided support and offered solutions.

A diagnosis of gestational diabetes (GD) means your blood glucose levels are too high. It is serious, and here's why: Moms who have GD often develop type 2 diabetes later in life if they do not make the necessary lifestyle changes. There is also a strong chance that you will have GD during future pregnancies, and therefore it has the possibility of changing your birth plan.

There are medical and natural options available to support you.

Once you have a plan for dealing with your gestational diabetes, should you be diagnosed, you should also include your birth team. For example, that could be your OBGYN, doula, nutritionist, midwife, and endocrinologist.

Also, it is important to know that the risks from gestational diabetes do not end at delivery. What you decide to do postpartum is also super important. Often this is the area that is not discussed and it is one of the most important aspects of your blood sugar handling plan, as it affects your and your baby's future health.

So What Is Gestational Diabetes?

According to babycenter.com[1], gestational diabetes is a form of diabetes that between 2 and 10 percent of expectant mothers can develop during pregnancy. These numbers are on the rise.

Hormonal changes during pregnancy affect the whole endocrine system. Those changes can cause a weak organ or gland to become out of balance. In the case of gestational diabetes, the weak gland would be the pancreas.

Normally, your body breaks down the sugars and carbohydrates you eat into a special sugar called glucose. Glucose fuels the cells in your body. A hormone called insulin produced in the pancreas then takes glucose from the bloodstream into the cells to be used as energy, or if not used, it is stored as fat.

If your pancreas can't produce enough insulin to keep up with your body's demand, you can have too much glucose in your bloodstream and therefore develop gestational diabetes.

Certain factors may lead to a higher risk for developing gestational diabetes. They are:

---

[1] "Gestational Diabetes," Baby Center, 2016, accessed May 18, 2017.

1. You are overweight prior to pregnancy and have a high BMI (body mass index) of greater than 25.

2. A diagnosis of gestational diabetes in previous pregnancies.

3. The presence of sugar in your urine or a family history of diabetes.

4. Excessive first-trimester weight gain

5. A poor diet has also been linked with a higher occurrence of gestational diabetes.

6. Hormone disruption. Perhaps you have a history of polycystic ovarian syndrome (PCOS) or autoimmune thyroid (Hashimoto's thyroiditis) or insulin resistance or hypoglycemia.

It is, however, possible to develop gestational diabetes without the presence of any of these risk factors. This is why most practitioners screen all of their patients between twenty-four and twenty-eight weeks of pregnancy.

How Gestational Diabetes Affects Your Baby

If you have gestational diabetes and your blood sugar levels are too high, your baby's blood sugar levels will also be too high. This will cause the baby's pancreas to produce more and more insulin, which can cause your baby to gain too much weight in utero.

As I mentioned earlier, big babies mean big shoulders and therefore an increased risk for the possibility of shoulder dystocia during the birthing process. A big baby also means that your baby is often too large to fit through the birth canal. This will mean a scheduled Caesarean Birth in 95 percent of cases.

If you have gestational diabetes your OBGYN will monitor the size of your baby and often schedule an early delivery via Caesarean

Birth. This should be motivation enough to want you to keep your weight and blood sugar under control.

Research has shown that babies born vaginally have stronger immune systems. A stronger immune system means a healthier baby.

On top of that, babies who are born with a higher than normal birth weight because of gestational diabetes often become overweight in childhood and adulthood, which can lead to other physical and emotional issues.

The Glucose Challenge Screening Test

No preparation is required prior to this test, and it is usually scheduled between twenty-six and twenty-eight weeks' gestation. During the test, you will be asked to drink a sweet liquid (glucose) and then will have blood drawn one hour after having the drink. This is when blood glucose levels normally peak and provide a reading that tells the doctor how well your body handles sugar. No fasting is required prior to this test.

A high level of glucose in your blood may indicate your body is not processing sugar effectively. This is a positive test. It is important to note that not all women who test positive for the glucose challenge screening are found to have gestational diabetes upon further diagnosis.

What Is in the Glucose liquid?

Ingredients: purified water, 50g dextrose (D-glucose derived from corn), citric acid, natural and artificial flavors, sodium benzoate, 0.1%, FD&C Yellow #6. It is also labeled "gluten free & dairy free.

What Happens Next If I Fail the Test?

Your doctor will want to schedule you for a follow-up test called the **glucose tolerance test** (which we describe in detail a little later in the chapter). The good news is you have some options available.

Not all moms that take the glucose challenge test are overweight. Some are following a paleo diet or low carb diet and therefore the sugary drink given at the glucose challenge test will cause a spike in blood sugar levels that the body is not used to.

There are also moms out there who are not doing a good job of managing their blood glucose on a day-to-day basis. Those moms are often hypoglycemic (have low blood sugar) or follow a vegetarian or vegan diet (too many carbs and not enough protein and veggies). Then there are moms who have had hormonal issues in the past or who are currently under high stress, that also fail the test.

This is a very good time to learn about your unique makeup and what foods, drinks, stressors, etc., affect your blood sugar levels. In some folks, a seemingly benign type of food can cause an increase in glucose levels. Examples I have seen are chicken, salmon, oranges, tomatoes, peanuts, and rice.

If you failed the glucose challenge test, this is like the check engine light coming on and telling you, "Hey, you need to make changes." Everyone has a unique profile, and this is where we can help understand your triggers.

Getting Blood Glucose under Control

We suggest that you follow these four steps if you failed the glucose challenge test, so you can learn more about how to manage your blood sugar.

First, if you are eating and drinking sugar and sweets, it is time to stop. Increase your intake of whole foods, in particular **VEGGIES**, and make sure you are getting adequate amounts of protein and good fats.

Second, get yourself a glucose monitor and some glucose strips so you can monitor your blood glucose levels.

Monitors and strips can be purchased through amazon.com, or they can be found in most pharmacies.

The glucose monitor and the strips come with instructions that are easy to follow. You will test your blood several times a day. While this is a lot of work the results will provide you with lots of good knowledge about how your body responds to certain foods and situations.

Interval	Range	Your Reading	Notes
Fasting, first thing in the morning	Less than 86mg/dl		
One hour after a meal	Less than 140mg/dl		
Two hours	Less than 125mg/dl		
Three hours	Back to fasting level less than 86mg/dl		

These levels are based on functional levels. The American Diabetic Association levels are slightly higher. There can be some variation, but the majority of readings should be in these ranges.

Third, start a blood sugar/food diary and record what you eat along with your glucose readings. By doing this you can then see clearly what foods or drinks cause higher spikes for you personally and which foods don't affect it as much or at all. Do this for ten to fourteen days.

If you start to see a trend of high sugars in the first couple of days, start modifying your diet. Make sure you are getting a balance of good protein, fat, and low glycemic carbs and see how these changes have an impact on the glucose values.

You'll probably also notice that there are many other factors that can affect you blood sugar levels. These are things like stress or lack of sleep.

Certain medications can also have an impact on your blood sugar levels. Other things like **EXERCISE** have a positive impact on maintaining normal blood glucose levels.

So if you're not exercising, it's time to get out there!

Fourth, once you have completed your ten to fourteen day food and blood sugar diary, take it to your OBGYN. If the numbers are consistently within range, then chances are high they will waive further testing. This is a huge bonus for most moms out there.

This of course does not mean that you run out and start eating poorly.

This is a huge wakeup call for you that you could be doing better with glycemic control, and the information you learned from your diary has high value. Going forward this could be the start of a healthier lifestyle for you and your family.

NOTE: Make sure you continue to ask your doctor to monitor the size of your baby because a big baby could alter the birth plan.

If you failed the glucose challenge test and you are still not able to get your blood sugar levels under control by following the steps we suggested, then your doctor would schedule you for a glucose tolerance test.

The Glucose Tolerance Test

Prior to taking the glucose tolerance test, your doctor will ask you to eat at least 150 grams of carbohydrates (about what you will get from a slice or two of whole grain bread, fruit, and sweet potatoes) for three days prior to taking the test. Then you will be required to fast.

You will not be permitted to eat or drink anything but sips of water for fourteen hours prior to the test. It is best to schedule the test for first thing in the morning.

Additionally, you should plan to have someone drive you to and from the test. Your energy levels may be low, and there is a slight possibility you may feel lightheaded.

When you arrive, the technician will draw blood to measure your baseline "fasting blood glucose level." You will be asked to drink a larger volume (or more concentrated solution) of the glucose drink than was used in the initial glucose challenge screening test. Your blood will be drawn and tested every hour for the next three hours.

The following are the values the American Diabetes Association considers to be abnormal during the glucose tolerance test: These are the levels used to diagnose gestational diabetes.

Functionally we like to see lower levels as mentioned above.

Interval	An Abnormal Reading	Your Reading	Notes
Fasting, first thing in the morning	Less than 95mg/dl		
One hour after a meal	Less than 180mg/dl		
Two Hours	Less than 155mg/dl		
Three hours	Less than 140mg/dl		

What if My Glucose Tolerance Test Results Are Abnormal?

If only one of your readings comes back abnormal, your doctor may suggest some changes to your diet and/or test you again later in the pregnancy.

If two or more of your readings come back abnormal, you'll be diagnosed with gestational diabetes and your doctor or midwife will recommend a treatment plan. Treating diabetes during pregnancy is extremely important! It is vital to protect the health of both mother and baby.

Going through the process of the glucose tolerance test is very stressful, so it is more important than ever that you stay positive and don't beat yourself up. Stay focused and breathe.

In most cases, gestational diabetes can be managed through eating a balanced, whole food diet, avoiding sugary processed foods like candy, cake, fast food and pretty much anything in a box. Plus getting some form of exercise every day should keep gestational diabetes under control. There are also certain supplements that can be helpful.

Now is the time to make the healthy diet changes if you want to have a healthy pregnancy and healthy baby. Changes you make now toward a healthier life will reap huge benefits for you, your baby, and your family going forward.

Again, as we said, don't beat yourself up about this setback, but see this as an opportunity to take control of how you see the future for you and your family.

If your levels remain high even with diet changes, supplementation, and regular exercise, then your doctor may prescribe medication.

If this happens your number one goal should be to continue to eat well, exercise, and above all enjoy the rest of your pregnancy.

What Is the Difference between Gestational Diabetes and Diabetes?

The Future

Although gestational diabetes often goes away with the birth of your baby, you still have to be aware of your increased risk of type 2 diabetes and take the necessary steps to prevent it.

Moms are very motivated during their pregnancy and outcomes are good. The key is to stay on track after baby is born. Moms who had gestational diabetes with their first pregnancy are much more likely to have gestational diabetes with their next pregnancy if they do not make permanent lifestyle changes.

Get screened. You should get the following tests six weeks to three months after delivery.

The tests are:

- Fasting glucose
- Hemoglobin A1C
- Insulin
- Full lipid panel, including triglycerides
- Liver panel

Then get checked every one or two years. By getting tested regularly, you will know when your blood sugar levels rise above normal (pre-diabetes) so you can take action before type 2 diabetes develops.

Maintaining a Healthy Weight

Being obese or overweight is one of the leading risk factors for developing type 2 diabetes. Even losing 5 to 10 percent of your body weight can dramatically cut your risk of developing type 2 diabetes. Your first goal should be to return to your pre-pregnancy weight by the time the baby is three to six months old.

Breastfeed your baby. This will help you lose weight. It's also been shown to reduce the risk of diabetes and obesity in your child.

Eat a healthy diet. Choose lean proteins, lots of veggies, leafy greens, good fats, nuts and seeds, some fruit, and a little whole grain. (See the back section of the book for Dr. Pia's Plant-Based Paleo Diet)

Move for at least thirty minutes a day. Whether you take a long walk, do yoga, or get your merengue groove on at a Latin dance class. Make it fun and a regular part of your day.

If you had gestational diabetes, your children are at risk for developing type 2 diabetes. Making changes to reduce your own risk can have a big impact on your kids.

Babies watch their parents' behavior and respond to situations and react to them. If your behaviors are healthy, then there is a good chance your children will follow your lead.

Dealing with Heartburn

Heartburn is caused by the contents of the stomach backing up via the esophageal sphincter. The major cause of this problem is that you are not digesting your food well. Therefore it is putrefying in the stomach and irritating the sphincter.

The sphincter can be irritated by certain foods, the extra pressure of the growing belly, a lack of stomach acid, or additional stress.

Digestion is best supported when your body is in parasympathetic mode.

Under stress the body is in sympathetic mode, which means all the blood from the central organs goes to extremities, and hydrochloric acid production in the stomach shuts down. What you want to do is make sure that when you eat you take a few minutes to relax and breathe. Optimal digestion occurs when the body is in parasympathetic mode. That is why it is often called "rest and digest."

It is also helpful to speak to your healthcare practitioner to see if adding some digestive enzymes or HCL (hydrochloric acid) support will help relieve your symptoms. You could also take a two-ounce shot of apple cider vinegar before each meal to stimulate stomach acid production.

We do not recommend the use of antacids and proton pump inhibitors like Pepcid because they make the overall problem worse and can cause other problems down the road. They treat the symptoms and not the root cause, which as we discussed is usually NOT enough stomach acid.

It could also be that you need to add more calcium to your diet. Calcium and HCL work together in the stomach to provide the optimal pH for digestion and for maintaining a healthy immune system. (Bacteria, viruses, and pathogens like E. coli, etc., cannot live in an acidic environment, so optimal pH in the stomach is important for overall health.)

Enjoying smaller meals more often could also be beneficial as can avoiding possible triggers such as spicy foods or foods that are made with bad fats.

The higher your BMI (body mass index) the higher the possibility of heartburn.

If you suspect you have a stomach ulcer then take action and visit your healthcare practitioner to discuss natural solutions.

How to Avoid Constipation?

Constipation is uncomfortable, and not only that, but also if one of your primary elimination processes is not working well it means toxins stay inside your body for too long. This can cause immune problems.

There are a number of things that could be the cause of your constipation challenges.

It could be the lack of fiber in your diet, so make sure you are getting enough—yet another great reason to increase the intake of your veggies and greens. If you have not already done so add our Ultimate Protein Smoothie to your diet and be sure to add the suggested fiber options.

You could be dehydrated. As discussed in earlier chapters, pregnant moms need lots of water.

It could be due to a lack of exercise. Exercise keeps all the fluids in the body moving well, and it also massages the internal organs of the digestive tract.

It could be that you are not digesting your foods well, and therefore foods are not broken down and absorbed. These undigested foods enter the digestive tract like a log and have a hard time passing through.

Digestive enzyme support could be helpful along with additional HCL (hydrochloric acid).

Some iron supplements can cause constipation, and for that reason we recommend food sources of iron like almonds, kelp, spinach, and grass-fed meats to help keep iron levels up. Iron also needs vitamin C to be absorbed well. If you do need to supplement iron, then we like a liquid formula called Floradix. For additional vitamin C add lemon or lime to your water.

You could be having thyroid problems. The thyroid controls the function of your basal metabolic rate. If the thyroid is "hypo" your basal metabolic rate will be slow and therefore so will the rate of digestion, absorption, and elimination.

Pregnancy is a time when hormones can fluctuate a lot. The endocrine glands like the thyroid are all linked together via a positive and negative feedback system, so when one gland is hyper (too fast) or hypo it can affect the others. If you suspect you are having issues with your thyroid, please check with your healthcare provider ASAP. The most common cause of miscarriage is linked to thyroid fluctuations.

It is also possible that you might have an imbalance in your gut flora. Taking a good probiotic at night before bed will help rebalance the gut.

If you have addressed all of the above and you are still having problems, add a magnesium supplement to the probiotic at night.

Magnesium is the co-factor for over three hundred enzymatic functions in the body, and it also acts as a muscle relaxer.

Why Do I Have Hemorrhoids and Varicose Veins?

These two seemingly unrelated issues have a common denominator. They are caused by venous congestion, usually of the hepatic portal vein. (Hepatic means relating to the liver.) The hepatic portal vein is a blood vessel that sends nutrient-rich blood from the gastrointestinal tract and spleen to the liver.

The liver is truly unique in how it receives its blood supply. Nearly every tissue and organ in the body receives nourishment and oxygen from blood delivered through an artery, which then carries blood under high pressure due to the heart's pumping action, through the body.

The liver, however, is the only organ to receive the majority of its blood supply through a large vein. This vein is called the portal vein. Why would the liver work this way? The pressure in veins, including the portal vein, is much lower than in arteries. The reduced pressure allows blood to percolate through the liver, which gives the liver's cells the time they need to do their primary work of detoxification.

Increased portal vein pressure—known medically as portal hypertension—causes blood to back up in the organs that send blood to the liver. The body tries to relieve the pressure by generating new blood vessels that bypass the blockage, but such vessels are often weak and twisted, and tend to bleed easily. These vessels are called varicose (varicose veins).

The liver, spleen, and intestines work overtime when a woman is pregnant. Rapid hormonal and weight changes can add additional stress to the liver. Once again, and I sound like a broken record, a good, healthy balanced diet, exercise, and optimal BMI are the best solutions.

If you do experience issues, then we have found that Collinsonia root works really well to support the venous system and therefore reduces hemorrhoids and varicose veins.

About Preeclampsia

Preeclampsia is a disorder that occurs only during pregnancy and the postpartum period. Preeclampsia affects both the mother and the unborn baby and occurs in at least 5–8 percent of all pregnancies.

Preeclampsia is a rapidly progressive condition characterized by high blood pressure and the presence of protein in the urine. Swelling, sudden weight gain, headaches, and changes in vision are important symptoms; however, some women with rapidly advancing disease report few symptoms.

Typically, preeclampsia occurs after twenty weeks gestation (in the late second or third trimesters or middle to late pregnancy) and up to six weeks postpartum (after delivery). In rare cases it can occur earlier than twenty weeks. Proper prenatal care is essential for diagnosing and managing preeclampsia.

Women who gain a lot of weight during pregnancy and eat foods that are high in sugar and bad fats have the highest risk of developing preeclampsia. As discussed, keeping a healthy whole-food diet is key.

If your blood pressure does start to climb, cut out all processed and packaged foods and make sure when you eat out that you choose healthy options. In some cases, additional calcium has been shown to be beneficial. High blood pressure can also be secondary to poor kidney function and high stress. Talk to your doctor if you experience any of the symptoms mentioned above.

Treating Anemia

The body needs iron to make hemoglobin, the molecule that is needed for the body to carry oxygen in the blood. Pregnant women need a lot of iron due to the fact that their red blood cell count increases 30 percent during pregnancy.

The biggest increase in blood volume happens in the third trimester and it's usually when your OBGYN will order a blood test to check for anemia. If you have been eating iron rich foods pre-conception and up until the third trimester you should have the stores you need. If you are diagnosed with anemia, then you will need to take an iron supplement.

We like organic sources of iron so you do not have problems absorbing and digesting iron, as this can result in unwanted symptoms like nausea and constipation. If you are taking supplemental iron, then you will need to also take it with vitamin C, which will assist with absorption.

We suggest liquid Floradix to our patients. Animal protein contains heme iron, which is the most bioavailable source of iron for the body. You can also obtain iron from non-heme sources, which come from plants. If you are vegan, vegetarian, experience heavy periods, or have a history of anemia, then we suggest getting tested earlier in the pregnancy to ensure you have adequate iron and are not anemic.

Here's a little tip: if you are feeling like you can't get your breath it could be a sign of air hunger, which can either mean you need iron-rich foods or antioxidants.

How Do I Overcome Stress and Have the Birth I Want?

We live in a non-stop always on 24/7 kind of world today. Everything is go, go, go, and we are bombarded with all kinds of interruptions and stimuli from text messages, Facebook posts, email, Snapchat, Instagram, and more. We rarely take the time out to just be with ourselves, be quiet, just breathe and relax. In many cases we do not know how.

How a person handles stress is personal, and that is why this is the most challenging part of your pregnancy. Staying in balance and harmony is difficult, let alone when you are pregnant, which in itself is stressful.

Here's how it works. When the body is under stress, cortisol levels rise. That's a good thing if we want to run away from the tiger, but if cortisol levels remain high for an extended period it can cause harm to your health.

When cortisol remains high it causes inflammation, which has a huge impact on the body. The body tries to do its best to shunt other calming or anti-inflammatory hormones to the stress-handling pathway to dampen down these high levels of cortisol. If the stress levels remain high, then over time imbalances occur in other hormones in the endocrine system. Usually this means higher than normal levels of circulating estrogen, or changes in testosterone can be the result.

Female bodies are amazing and they were made to give birth to babies. Tapping in to all the things you have learned in the book will support you when the times comes for your baby to arrive.

78

The Best Way to Think about Stress and Your Unborn Child

Some anxious moms feel really good in their third trimester. They say they've never felt better. Why is that? The answer is that Mom is taking adrenal support from her baby. What happens next is, baby's adrenal glands are depleted and more often than not baby has a tendency to be sensitive, have sleep issues, or be anxious, fussy, suffer from ADHD, and the like. We see this a lot in children who were the first born in their family, and particularly if they were the first born after a previous miscarriage.

We are learning more and more that the womb is not a sterile environment and that Mom's environment (mind, body, and spirit) has a direct effect on the environment of baby in the womb.

Keeping stress low during pregnancy will be beneficial for Mom and baby. This is where Dad can play a big role along with other members of your support team.

If you have been following along with us you know that choosing to follow a path of healthy eating, exercise, sleep, etc., all lower the levels of cortisol in the body and therefore make it much easier to have a nurturing mindset, which is good for Mom and baby. http://www.headspace.com

Getting out and in touch with nature or deep breathing exercises are also great stress relievers. For me personally, I enjoy yoga, a walk along the beach, planting a garden, and dinner with good friends. These are all good stress relievers for me.

I strongly suggest you find what works for you and practice it often throughout your pregnancy and your life.

It won't mean that you will not have stressful situations; however, you will be better equipped to handle them.

Chapter 6

THE FOURTH TRIMESTER: CONGRATULATIONS! YOU HAVE A NEW BABY!

The moment a child is born, the mother is also born. She never existed before. The woman existed, but the mother never. A mother is something absolutely new.

—Rajneesh

Congratulations on the birth of your baby!

I have been lucky enough to be able to be in the room after a birth on several occasions. The energy, wonder, and love that flows between Mom, Dad, and their new baby is like nothing else I have ever experienced. It is like being in a dreamland and something powerful has just taken place—and in fact, it has! You are holding a human that has a piece of your genic blueprint and a piece of your partner's genic blueprint.

I truly hope you had a gentle and beautiful birth. I hope it was what you wanted for yourself and your child. If not, then that is OK and it is time to move forward with the healing process. Birth is exhilarating and stressful at the same time. It takes a lot of energy, so hopefully you have taken some time to cocoon as a family.

If you have been following along with us, then you have healthy practices in place and your resilience factor should be high and the healing process much quicker.

Having some things in place prior to birth can be helpful. Making sure you have some healthy foods stocked away in the freezer, engaging the help of a food service, or hiring a postpartum doula are some of the things we suggest. This will allow you the time you all need to rest and recoup and settle into a sleep, wake, feed routine with your new baby.

Bouncing Back after Birth

It is normal to feel a little of the baby blues after giving birth. During pregnancy your placenta has guided your endocrine system to increase progesterone levels to a higher level than you might have experienced before. Some moms tell me they only feel really great when they are pregnant. Progesterone is the feel-good, calming hormone, and once you have given birth and the placenta has been removed, your hormone level of progesterone drops. This abrupt drop can take a little adjustment.

Some women choose to have their placentas encapsulated. This is a process where the placenta is removed and dried and put into capsule form. The idea is that you take these capsules postpartum.

This process has been shown to help moms combat the baby blues.

For more information, we suggest you talk to your doula, midwife, or healthcare provider. Do your research to ensure this is the right decision for you.

If you had a Caesarean Birth, we suggest you treat this as a recovery from major surgery. You will need to detox the drugs and antibiotics and support tissue healing.

To do that, we suggest adding a proteolytic enzyme to your diet to support tissue healing. These enzymes taken away from food will help significantly with recovery and act as an anti-inflammatory.

Continue with your probiotics to support healthy gut flora following a course of antibiotics, and in some cases you might need to increase your dose for a short time.

Make sure you drink plenty of clean water, not only to flush out toxins and tissue damage but also to encourage adequate milk supply. In some cases, you will want to increase your antioxidants like vitamin C for a short period of time to support healing.

Consider Arnica, a homeopathic remedy to help with internal bruising and trauma.

Lastly, continue to eat well to support the healing process and to provide your baby with healthy breast milk.

A special note: Resilience and the bounce factor are critical to a speedy recovery. If you are in good physical, nutritional, and emotional shape going into your pregnancy and you do have to have a Caesarean Birth, then the better and faster you will recover.

Foods that Support Lactation and Milk Production

Research shows us that breastfeeding is the very best option for your new baby. Study after study concludes that breastfed babies thrive and outperform on cognitive skill tests versus those babies that were bottle-fed.

Nature innately knows how to formulate the right nutrients your baby needs. We know that in today's world it is challenging to breastfeed your baby until they are naturally weaned. However, we strongly suggest you allow three months as the minimum amount of frame. The longer you can breastfeed, the better for your baby. We should also mention that the bonding that occurs between mom and baby during breastfeeding and the act of providing nourishment from one human to another couldn't be denied as anything other than very special.

Breast milk contains mother's colostrum, which is very high in antibodies. That along with a vaginal birth provides a jump-start to a strong immune system for your new baby.

Breast milk is also easier for your baby to digest than most of the common baby formulas, unless of course, you, mom, are eating foods that cause you or baby to have a histamine (allergic) response. Histamine is high when you are exposed to something the body sees as a pathogen. It triggers the inflammation cascade.

Typically, I have found that if moms eat a lot of processed foods like dairy or foods with soy, newborns can have digestive challenges trying to break down these proteins.

The symptoms that show up in your child are typically gas, bloating, digestive pain, and increased spit-ups, etc. In some cases, we have added digestive support for Mom so she can break down the proteins and therefore baby's digestive problems are resolved. If not, then it is best to do an elimination diet and avoid all dairy and soy to see if the problem resolves itself.

If not, then please check in with your lactation consultant http://www.mamasandmilk.com or your pediatrician.

Jane's Story

Jane was two months old when she came in to see me. She was having challenges with her digestion. Mom was breastfeeding, and baby Jane was not keeping her food down. She was spitting up, crying a lot, and not gaining weight. Mom was also very sure that baby Jane was having pain associated with her digestive challenges. Mom was beside herself with worry, and baby Jane was on Zantac, an acid reflux medication.

We performed an exam on baby and mom and learned that mom had had a bout of diarrhea and baby Jane was having challenges digesting proteins (soy and dairy). We gave mom a natural supplement to soothe her digestive tract, and ask her to take soy and dairy of her diet. We also discussed how stress hormones and high cortisol could have an impact on baby Jane via the breast milk. Baby Jane and mom came in a week later for a follow up, and mom reported that baby was off all medications, was feeding well, and was calm and gaining weight. Mom was also feeling a lot better.

Hopefully you have been following our healthy eating guidelines for pregnancy so your milk supply will be rich in nutrients. You should continue going down this path, making sure you are consuming adequate quantities of good fats and lots of filtered water. We also suggest continuing on your omega-3 fatty acid supplementation. If you are struggling with milk production, adding fenugreek has also been shown to be beneficial.

Most moms who breastfeed could feel even hungrier than when they were pregnant, as breastfeeding burns up to five hundred calories per day.

This is also a time when some moms and dads abandon their balanced and beautiful pregnancy diet and start sneaking those not-so-good-for-you foods back into their meal plans. Remember, what you eat, drink, and think, your baby does too. This is especially true if you are breastfeeding your baby.

How Does Diet Affect Breast Milk

Your own diet has an impact on your breast milk. Breast milk can taste and smell different at each feeding based on what you have consumed. Your baby is being exposed to all the different flavors you eat and drink through your breast milk. Baby will particularly notice if you had a spicy meal, as they will be consuming the spice too.

If you experience challenges with breastfeeding, we recommend you contact a lactation consultant. They are experts and will be able to provide information and resources to help support you through this new experience.

We have talked about all the benefits of breastfeeding; however, in some cases breastfeeding is not possible, so we suggest you don't stress, and look for milk formula options that do not contain SOY.

We like a recipe derived from the Weston Price Foundation. Dave Asprey, who is a published nutrition expert and author of the Better Baby Book, also recommends this recipe.

Formula Recipe:

- 1 cup of milk-based powdered formula (Nutramigen or Alimentum)
- 29 oz. of filtered water
- 1 large raw organic egg yolk
- ½ teaspoon of cod liver oil
- Raw organic cream
- 1 teaspoon of pure oil (sunflower, walnut, sesame [rotate oils])
- 1 teaspoon of MCT (medium-chain triglyceride) oil

1. Blend thoroughly and refrigerate. When heating put the bottle in hot water and do not overheat, as the formula will denature.

2. There are goat milk based recipes available if your baby does not tolerate whey.

Taking Probiotics While I am Breastfeeding

Yes you can. Taking probiotics is especially important if you had a Caesarean Birth or IV antibiotics due to GBS (group B strep). In some cases, we have suggested a probiotic for baby in addition to one for mom. In this case it is typically when the birth has been difficult and there has been the need for surgery or additional antibiotic medication.

We have also suggested additional probiotics for babies who have come to us having experienced immune challenges and are having difficulty with feeding and absorbing nutrients.

There are some great baby probiotic formulas out there; however, we like to use mom's probiotic. Simply break open the capsule and put a little bit on your finger and have baby suck it off your finger. That way baby can absorb the probiotic quickly. It can begin to work and does not taste bad.

Continuing Prenatal Vitamins

We suggest you continue to eat well, consuming a variety of whole nutritious foods, and continue to take your prenatal supplements for at least three months and then switch over to my Fab Five.

The Fab Five is well rounded and covers a lot of health and wellness bases. Together with a good diet they can keep you healthy. At a minimum we recommend taking the following supplements every day: probiotic, fish oil, a B-complex, a mineral supplement, and a digestive enzyme. Here's why:

1. Probiotics

Probiotics support healthy gut flora, maintain a healthy gut environment, and improve nutrient digestion and absorption. They support GI immune health and are a good **adjunct to antibiotic** therapy, which has been overprescribed for years. Probiotics are best taken at night, as this is when your digestive system does its work.

2. Omega-3 Fatty Acids

Omega-3s are a good source of DHA and EPA essential fatty acids. These are called the GOOD Fats. Omega-3s act as an anti-inflammatory and support optimal cardiovascular function help keep blood stable and support brain health.

3. A B Vitamin Complex

B-complex vitamins help improve nerve conductivity, support blood sugar imbalances, and help with hypotension (low blood pressure) and drug and alcohol use. A lack of Vitamin B can lead to depression and anxiety. This is a must-have if you are a vegan or vegetarian, because you are not getting the most bioavailable for the body B vitamins from your diet.

4. A Mineral Supplement

For most of us, the best mineral supplement is in the form of a calcium-magnesium-vitamin D3 combo. In some cases zinc is the mineral that would be most beneficial.

5. Digestive Enzymes

For most of us, digestive enzymes are a combo of pepsin and hydrochloric acid (HCL). Stress reduces the production of HCL, and therefore we often suffer from digestive issues due to the body's inability to break down food.

Digestive enzymes help with indigestion, gas, and bloating. They also help with calcium, anemia, and iron absorption. If you have sour breath, they are a must.

Other than the Fab Five there is a possibility that you might need to increase your consumption of antioxidants like vitamin C, vitamin E, and vitamin A.

The need for iron decreases after birth, so we suggest you stop supplementing with iron and instead eat iron-rich foods. However, if you had a lot of blood loss during birth you should talk with your physician about having your iron levels checked.

If you have questions it is always prudent to check in with your health and wellness doctor for your unique needs.

Postpartum Weight Loss

If this were your first pregnancy you would no doubt expect that once you had your baby your belly bump would magically disappear. The truth is it can take a little while for the uterus and the increase in fluid volume during pregnancy to get back to normal.

You can expect about twelve plus pounds in weight loss the first week or two post-delivery.

The combination of the weight of baby, the placenta, amniotic fluid, and water and blood loss add up to about twelve plus pounds. If you have been following along with our plan you would have gained no more than twenty-five pounds. The way to look at this is that you have lost half your baby weight very quickly even though you still feel swollen and pregnant the first day or two after delivery.

The days following birth can be hectic as you, your family, and your baby establish the patterns for sleeping, eating, and living.

I always suggest that families take time during the first week to ten days to cocoon and establish rhythms that work for everyone in the family. There is a ton of information out there about how many feedings baby should be having, how much sleep, how much poop, how much weight should baby be gaining, etc.

Having a baby is not like having a wearable device like a Fitbit with beepers going off telling you when to do this and when to do that. Can they be helpful? Yes. However building a human is an organic process that requires mindful attention.

I must admit I am a little shocked at how popular the electronic baby changer pad has been. I am not sure I would expose my newborn child to the effects of EMF so I could monitor their every oz., poop, heart rate, etc., when there is still so much unknown about the effects

Once you and your family have established a routine that is best for you all, then it is time to get back on the exercise bandwagon.

Start with walking, which you and baby can do together, and then gradually increase the intensity and the amount. If you had a Caesarean Birth or other complications during birth, then it will take longer to recover and get back to a regular exercise routine. There are some wonderful resources available for you like FIT4MOM.com or post-natal mom and baby yoga classes.

If you choose to breastfeed your baby, you will also benefit from some additional weight loss.

The way to think about postpartum weight loss is this: **Am I eating the right amount of whole food nutrients so I can provide optimal nutrition through my breast milk for my baby?** If you do that your weight will balance out naturally.

This is not the time to put weight loss and possible dietary restrictions above nutrient-dense foods. When you balance your energy with the right amount of exercise and foods for you, you will never have to worry about weight gain. This rule applies whether you are pregnant or not.

Why is it Important to Take Care of Yourself First Then Baby?

This is the area where the wheels fall off for most new parents. They do a good job of staying fit and relatively healthy prior to having a family. Then the first baby comes along and they are now consumed 24/7 with the needs of the baby and they neglect the healthy behaviors they once had in place for themselves

Stress levels go up, sleep is almost always challenging, and slowly but surely that can lead to less-than-optimal diet choices.

Even the most grounded, well-informed moms and dads worry and stress over every detail in the first few weeks of their newborn's life. It is a natural instinct to nurture. However, if you find yourself over-obsessing and neglecting yourself, then take a step back and take some deep breaths and trust that all will be OK. Ask yourself what advice you would give to someone else.

What you don't want is to fast-forward a few years and the kids are now off to school and you find yourself 10/20/30 pounds overweight and feeling bad.

What happened? Where did the time go? The best thing for you and your family long-term is to make time to take care of yourself. Kids want parents that are full of vitality and energy. They need good role models so they too can grow up to be healthy and vital adults. I can't stress this enough.

You can't take care of others if you don't take care of yourself first.

You can't give to others if you are stressed out, tired, and overweight. Sit together as a family and make a plan so everyone will thrive.

Drinking Alcohol while Breastfeeding

The decision is yours. The research shows that drinking alcohol can inhibit lactation and in turn reduce your milk supply. If you are having challenges with milk production, then abstinence is the best course of action.

If you choose to drink, then do so right after a feed so your body has a chance to metabolize the alcohol. If you know you are going out to have a couple of drinks with friends, we suggest that you plan ahead and pump extra milk before consuming alcohol.

A note: The liver will detox alcohol first. So know that if you drink, your major organ of detoxification will be busy dealing with the alcohol.

Your Universe Is Baby's Universe; Baby's Universe Is Your Universe

We have talked a lot about the importance of diet, supplementation, and exercise. What we haven't yet discussed are the effects of a calm and loving environment on pregnancy, the birth, and the days and months following birth.

I have practiced yoga for almost all of my adult life, and my overall goal when I step into the yoga room is one of restoration of the mind, body, and spirit. This attention and intention has helped me through some challenging times and allows me to manage stress and stay focused and calm when treating my patients. We know that when we are in a loving, positive, and calm environment, we thrive. We also know that when we are in an environment that is toxic, filled with stress and anger, we either hunker down or lash out.

The same is true for your baby. When young parents come in to see me to seek help for an issue with baby, I always ask them about their environment first. This idea is the same as dealing with the root cause versus a symptom. If I have a pain, the question would be "What is my body trying to tell me?" versus let me take a pill to knock out the pain. The same goes for baby. What is my baby trying to tell me? To answer the question, you have to look holistically and consider baby's whole environment.

I was standing in the grocery line one day and a young baby was acting out, and the mom turned me and said out loud, "I don't know where he gets that from." It is one of the classic statements we have all heard before.

I know what I thought. What do you think? That's right. The baby learned that behavior or way of being from his environment.

92

A brand-new study published in October 2016 in the journal Science, led by Mercedes Pardes of the University of California, San Francisco, https://www.researchgate.net/publication/309258278_Extensive_migration_of_young_neurons_into_the_infant_human_frontal_lobe further supports that our early interactions with babies might establish long-lasting effects on behavior. This study suggests that babies' frontal lobe neurons are not fully developed until they are four to six months old. The study suggests that there is brain development outside the womb in the fourth trimester.

I often have the joy of treating moms who are newly pregnant through to postpartum and beyond. When they bring their newborn baby in for their first checkup after the birth, the babies already know me and respond to me. They know my voice. Moms are always surprised, and it is a true joy for me.

As you go through the process of parenting from pre-conception though birth and beyond give the idea of a holistic, mindful environment some good thought.

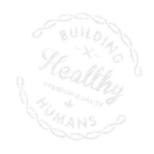

Chapter 7
BRINGING IT ALL TOGETHER

Imagine what might happen if women emerged from
their labor beds with a renewed sense of the strength and
power of their bodies and of their capacity for ecstasy
through giving birth.

—Christiane Northrup

The Best Gift You Can Give Your Child

We hope we have answered most of the questions that arise when
you are thinking about having a baby, or are currently pregnant and
looking for what is best for you and your baby.

We also hope we have answered some of your concerns and
challenges if you are postpartum and currently breastfeeding
your baby.

We hope we did this in a straightforward and easy-to-understand
format. That was our goal. We didn't want to decide your choices
for you; we wanted you and your family to be informed to be able
to think about the choices you make and then consciously decide
what is best for you all.

We wanted you to understand that having a balanced and beautiful
pregnancy and a happy, healthy baby is all about the choices that

you as parents or soon-to-be parents make each and every day. If what I said connected with you, then I know future generations will benefit from your attention and care, not only now, but also for the rest of their lives.

It's not about being perfect, which is very stressful, by the way. It's about being mindful and living in the moment. I know groundbreaking technologies will continue to try to make our lives longer and easier. However, what I hope is that what you take away from this book is that our lives also need to have balance and quality.

You need to get back to simple principals like whole, unprocessed foods, clean water, being in nature, having a sense of community, and exercise. These principals and actions are necessary to offset our 24/7 high-tech world.

If you want future generations to have a high quality of life, then you are called to do your part. It is our responsibility as parents to guide our children to make healthy life choices and for them to continue those practices with their children.

Today's technology via the study of epigenetics has confirmed that those simple experiments Dr. Pottenger conducted so many years ago on the cats are right, and what you eat, drink, and think has a long-lasting impact on our offspring and future generations. For your very own organic handmade Pottenger Cat. Go to http://palmsprout.etsy.com

Thank you so much for reading this book. It has been a labor of love for me to take this long-held idea and put it into words.

I hope what I have said changes the way you think about the future, and I also hope you share this message with family and friends.

Namaste!

Resources
THE P21 PROGRAM

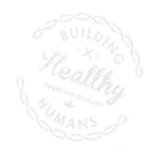

INTRODUCTION

The P21 Program is a purification program designed specifically for soon to be pregnant moms and dads who want to have a happy healthy baby.

Preparing for pregnancy is not something we talk about a lot and we certainly keep things under wraps if we are struggling to get pregnant. It's a huge life transition and like most transitions it requires some conscious thought, planning and preparation.

Things are quite different than they were decades ago. Today women often-live stressful work intensive lives that require that we take a moment and think about what we want (a happy healthy baby) before we decide to get pregnant. You owe it to yourself to prepare, feel empowered and be ready for the changes ahead.

One of the best things you and your partner can do is prepare your bodies nutritionally so that you can give yourselves and your unborn child the very best start.

This program will most probably require you to make some changes to your current diet and lifestyle. For some of you that might mean you need to give up (not choose) your favorite foods. For some of you this will be more of an emotional challenge than a physical one. Many of our life stories and memories are centered on emotional attachments to certain foods and behaviors.

The truth is that within a matter of days of beginning the P21 program you will start to feel lighter, stronger and have more energy. Sleep will improve, as will some of those annoying issues like bloating, allergies, PMS, headaches and more. You will start to have a greater sense of wellbeing. For some of you it will be the first time in ages that you have actually felt this good.

One last thing before you start. Keep everything in perspective.

Getting your nutritional house in order will also give you a greater sense of clarity into your physical and emotional wellbeing, however it is also important to listen to yourself and love yourself so that you can prepare to become a conscious parent.

Why should you do P21 program before conception and why is it important?

Here is why.

At one time eating a "healthy diet" and making sure you're taking the right dose of methylfolate was all that was needed. However in the past decade we've seen an escalation in health conditions that affect kids,

These include allergies (including food and environmental) to asthma, eczema, autoimmune diseases and the list goes on... We have also seen a massive rise in the number of kids with autism. Many of these conditions can be traced back to environmental toxin exposure of one or more of the parents of these kids.

These toxic exposures can affect fertility and the genes we express, which then get passed on to our babies at the time of conception.

Quite frankly I am scared to death that if we do not take back our health now and teach our children how to enjoy real foods that are found in nature we are heading for higher and higher medical costs, higher obesity rates, and a generation of children that will not outlive their parents

If you have taken the time to read this far you know we think that providing good building blocks for your soon to be born baby is essential.

We suggest that you and your partner do the P21 program together 3-6 months prior to conception. Then follow a modified maintenance version of the program to be sure you continue healing and have optimal health at the time of conception. If you are struggling with Infertility the P21 program is a must do first step.

If you and your partner live or work in environments where you are exposed to toxic chemicals or metals then the P21 detox is also a must!

If you have any health conditions we suggest that you seek help and work with someone who knows the best way to support you while you go through the program.

What is Purification?

"It's Nutritional Boot Camp for Your Body, Mind and Spirit."

Purification is the internal cleansing and detoxification of your body. Think of it as "spring cleaning" for your insides. It requires making new and healthier choices for yourself. You will be discontinuing fast foods, processed convenience foods, and sugar-laden snacks.

These foods place an unnecessary load on your body and provide little or no nutrients.

During your 21 day journey you will experience the healing power of whole unprocessed, preservative free foods, lots of pure spring water, tasty fresh fruit, lots of vegetables, healing greens and delicious protein loaded shakes. We also include Dr. Pia recommended daily supplement plan that is designed to support and heal your organs.

In some special cases we will make adjustments to the program based on your unique needs.

You will also receive daily emails that provide coaching and lifestyle support during this transformational journey.

You will begin to realize just how much food you unconsciously snack on throughout the day. We have become a society of snackers. Did that one cookie or that handful of chips really count? We eat mindlessly throughout the day and then wonder why we put on weight and don't feel all that great.

The P21 program will help educate you on how to eat, how to listen to your body and become more mindful about the choices you make! You will shed some extra weight and rid yourself of accumulated sludge.

Look Great, Feel Great, Rejuvenate.

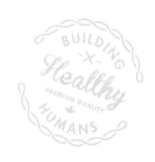

HOW IS THE P21 PROGRAM DIFFERENT?

This program is designed to help you learn how to live a healthier life, by cleansing not only the colon but also detoxifying other vital organs like the liver, the kidneys, the lungs and the skin.

The use of whole food, and supportive supplements help you purify your body from the inside out. The P21 program teaches you how to nurture your body and provide it with the nutrients it needs to rejuvenate.

You will lose weight; you will feel light; all those aches and pains will be gone; your skin will glow; your eyes will sparkle with vitality; your sugar cravings will be diminished if not gone; your energy will skyrocket, and your whole attitude will be that of positivity, and you will know how to maintain those feelings of total well-being forever!

I believe that given the proper nutrition your body has the amazing capability for healing.

Food in the right combination is medicine to the body.

I also believe that nutrition should be individualized to meet each patient's needs, and health concerns. When needed we include additional Doctor recommended supplement products.

It is amazing to me to watch as patients start the program on Day 1 with some trepidation and then see them skip out of my office Day 21 feeling great and looking amazing. They are always astounded at the results and the P21 program always exceeds their expectations.

I have now conducted hundreds of P21 programs and have taken all of the knowledge I have learned from my patients and designed a program that is easy to follow, simple and extremely effective.

I want you all to have a beautiful and balance pregnancy and a happy healthy baby. This is the best way to start!

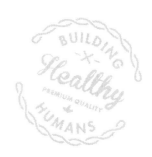

THE BEAUTY IS IN THE SIMPLICITY...

1. EAT LOTS OF VEGGIES AND SOME FRUITS

2. ENJOY A DELICIOUS PROTEIN PACKED SMOOTHIE

3. FOLLOW THE SIMPLE SUPPLEMENT ROUTINE

4. EXERCISE EACH DAY & DRINK LOTS OF WATER!

This is a whole body purification program. Much of the program centers on what you eat. The foundation of the P21 program includes eating whole organic and unprocessed foods, supporting the body with Dr. Pia recommended supplements and drinking plenty of water.

PLANNING IS THE KEY TO A SUCCESSFUL P21 PROGRAM

1. Take the time to read the instructions and think through your 3-week journey and what this means for you and for the future of your unborn child. There might be some modifications for some of you based on your health needs.

2. Get an updated physical and baseline labs to determine where you are right now.

3. Cut back on sugary foods, alcohol and caffeine the week before you start the P21 program. If you choose not to do that you may experience a good size headache as your body goes the through the withdrawal of sugar and caffeine. Not fun!

4. Plan your shopping list and think through the best way to prepare your meals. I like to do this on Sunday, so I am ready for the week ahead.

5. It's a good idea to chop your raw veggies and to lightly steam veggies like sweet potato, broccoli, Brussels sprouts etc. in advance and store in them fridge. That way you have them ready to go.

6. Clean up you Kitchen and clear your fridge and cupboards of tempting processed sugar laden foods. If it's not around you can't be tempted to eat it.

7. Make sure you eat enough of the allowed foods. The program is designed to keep your blood sugar stable. You should never be hungry.

8. The protein packed Shake is best made fresh however if you can't do that prepare the whole batch of shake in the morning and take the afternoon shake with you in a container to work with your veggies and fruit.

9. If possible refrain from social engagements were food is involved the first week of the P21 program. If that is impossible you should try to influence the choice of where you will either have lunch or dinner. Better yet have your family and friends over to your home and show them how to make tasty and good for you food.

10. If you do go out choose places where you know the food is high quality and fresh. Most places will accommodate a large plate of steamed veggies or a big salad with oil and vinegar dressing on the side. During week two you can include 3oz of protein.

11. Stick with your regular workout routine. It is good to sweat, however if you feel a little lethargic the first week while your body gets rid of all those built up toxins, talk a short walk or just relax and take some quite time to notice the changes that are happening. However get back on the exercise bandwagon Day 8.

12. Hopefully you and your partner are doing this as a family. If not then discuss the program and the guidelines with you partner. You will naturally become a little introspective especially the first week and they will need to understand this.

13. **This is the most important tip!** Once you have completed the P21 program, it is very important that you reintroduce foods one at a time. For example: many of us have sensitivities to processed wheat, dairy and soy products, so we want you to be mindful as you go through that process. You will want to observe the way your body reacts to different foods. The P21 program is just the start of a new healthier lifestyle for you and your family.

14. If you do choose to indulge in not so great food and drink after you have completed the P21 program, please understand that it could be a big challenge for your immune system. The impact could cause you to be susceptible to whatever malady is going around. After all the hard work you do not want that.

15. Enjoy the journey and take the time to reflect on all areas of your life. Congratulations on taking this step to do this for yourself

and your future child. You will look and feel amazing at the completion of this program and be have the building blocks in place to have a beautiful and balanced pregnancy and a happy healthy baby.

Donna's Experience

"Thanks for introducing me to The P21 Program. Not only is the process a wonderful program but also it's a wonderful program that works. My success on the program was a direct result of a well-planned organized program. I'm more then happy to share my results and success of the program so that others can be steps closer to a healthier life style. I would recommend the program to anyone because of the amazing results that the program has given me. Once again thank you Dr. Pia for your support and knowledge Please help as many people as you can with this wonderful program."

- Donna

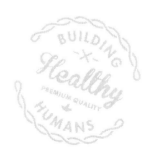

WHAT CAN YOU EAT?

Focus on what you can eat and about eating a variety of nutrient dense foods.

- Think about eating a rainbow of colors.
- Follow our suggested daily meal plan so you maintain your blood sugar levels and do not go hungry.
- Modifications should be made to your specific needs.

You can eat unlimited quantities of the vegetables on the list below. They should be fresh or frozen, organic raw or if needed lightly steamed. A stir-fry is also OK. **You should eat twice as many vegetables as fruit. I will say this again: You should eat twice as many veggies as fruit!**

VEGGIES

Artichokes	Cabbage
Arugula	Cauliflower
Asparagus	Carrots
Bamboo Shoots	Celery
Beets and Beet greens	Chicory/radicchio
Broccoli	Chives
Brussels Sprouts	Collard Greens
Boy Choy	Cucumbers
Black Radishes	Chard
Bell Peppers	Dandelion Greens
Bean Sprouts	Eggplant
Belgian Endive	Endive/escarole

Fennel

Hearts of Palm

Kale

Kohlrabies

Lettuce/ Leafy greens

Mushrooms

Mustard greens

Okra

Onions

Parsnips

Pumpkins

Radishes

Shallots

Spinach

Squash, all varieties

Sweet Potatoes (1/2 cup/day)

Turnips

Watercress

Water Chestnuts

Yucca roots

Zucchini

FRUIT

Use fresh, frozen and organic fruit if possible – Stick to a * low glycemic fruits with high fiber content as a mid morning snack otherwise only use fruit for your smoothies / shakes. Serving size (¾ cup)

*Apples

*Avocado

Apricots

*Blackberries

*Blueberries

Bananas -⅓ to ½
    per smoothie

Cantaloupe

Cherries

Clementine

*Coconuts

Cranberries

Figs

Grapes (15)

*Grapefruit

Guavas

Kiwis

Kumquats

*Lemons

*Limes

*Logan Berries

Melons

Mango

Mulberries

Nectarines	Pineapple
Oranges	Pomegranates
Olives	*Raspberries
Papayas	Rhubarb
*Pears	*Strawberries
Peaches	Tomatoes
Plums	Tangerines

PROTEIN

You will enjoy at least two Protein Packed Shakes per day.

Beginning on Day 11 you can add 3 ounces of additional protein to one meal per day. Choose Organic Free Range Chicken, Eggs or Wild Fresh Fish, which you can prepare by broiling, baking or poaching. If you are an athlete or have a physical occupation we then suggest including additional protein on Day 1 of the P21 program.

WATER

The rule of thumb is to drink ½ your body weight in ounces. If you are 128 pounds then you will drink 64 ounces of water a day minimum. The benefits of clean filtered water are numerous. Water keeps our cells hydrated AND supports healthy digestion and elimination.

FATS

You can use 4-7 teaspoons a day. Use only high quality cold pressed oils. Coconut Oil, Flaxseed Oil, Grape Seed Oil, Extra Virgin Olive Oil and Avocado.

HERBS AND SPICES

Herbs and Spices add flavor to your food and many of them are known for their anti-inflammatory and healing properties. I like to add Cilantro and parsley to a mixed green salad or sprinkle turmeric on veggies. If you have a sensitive digestive system or an autoimmune condition we suggest staying away from spices that cause irritations.

Basil	Mint
Bay Leaves	Mustard
Cardamom	Nutmeg
Cayenne	Oregano
Chili Powder	Paprika
Chives	Parsley
Cilantro	Pepper
Cinnamon	Rosemary
Cloves	Sage
Cumin	Sea Salt
Dill	Tarragon
Garlic	Thyme
Ginger	Turmeric
Lemon Grass	

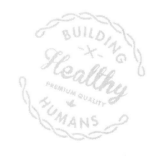

A SUPER SIMPLE DAILY MEAL PLAN

I like to keep things simple and easy! I also know that if the P21 Program is too complicated you will give it up and not enjoy the benefits of the full 21 days. For those of you who love to experiment this is a good place to start and for those of you who don't know where to start. Just do this:

Breakfast: "The Shake/Smoothie" and your morning Doctor recommended supplements. Choose one of the easy to follow Shake recipes on the following page.

Mid Morning: One piece of fruit from the suggested list. If you used a banana in the shake do not have another one – that is too much fruit sugar. Choose berries or an apple instead. Kale Chips are also a great nutrient dense snack.

One hour before Lunch: Set a timer so you don't forget. Take the supplements with a big glass of water. You should have had a least 3 glasses of water by now.

Lunch: Most of us need a lunch that is easy to eat, doesn't require tools and is easy to transport. Fill a large container with a variety of cut veggies that are raw or lightly steamed. (For example carrots, radishes, broccoli, cauliflower, and asparagus, celery etc.) Add a creamy avocado and herb/spice based dip

Mid Afternoon: Have your second "Shake/Smoothie" for the day. DON'T miss this shake. (If you are an athlete and have a strong workout program please discuss with Dr. Pia as we may want to add a third shake to the program).

One hour before Dinner: Again, set your timer. Take your supplements with a large glass of water.

Dinner: Grab a big bowl and fill it with mixed organic leafy greens. Add tomatoes, avocado, chopped sweet potatoes, beets, spring onions, and bell peppers etc. Dress the salad with one of the suggested salad dressing recipes. Don't soak you salad with too much dressing.

OR: Use a little sesame or coconut oil and lightly stir-fry you favorite veggies and spices. I like to alternate between a big salad bowl and a stir-fry for a little variety

Following this plan makes sure you get twice as many veggies as fruit and it is easy if you take the time to shop, chop and plan ahead of time.

ALL DAY: Drink water throughout the day. HINT: do not to drink too much after 6/7pm or you could find your self up at night.

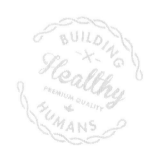

SAMPLE SHAKE RECIPES

THE TRUE FOOD BASIC SHAKE

- 1 - 1 ½ cups of frozen fruit or veggies
- 1 tbs of flaxseed oil
- 2 scoops of PROTIEN shake
- 1 tbs whole food fiber
- 8 ounces of water

Mix in a blender and enjoy! You can double this recipe so you have enough for your whole day. Keep Refrigerated.

PURE BERRY SHAKE

- ½ cup of frozen blueberries and ½ cup of frozen strawberries OR Raspberries
- ½ banana
- 1tbs of flaxseed oil
- 2 scoops of PROTIEN shake
- 1 tbs whole food fiber
- 8 ounces of water

(We like to add a handful of spinach to this one for added nutrients)

Mix in a blender and enjoy! You can double this recipe so you have enough for your whole day. Keep Refrigerated

So that you can have some fun experimenting we have included our Ultimate Protein Shake Recipe to use a guide

THE ULTIMATE PROTEIN SHAKE RECIPE

How to make the base for the Ultimate Protein Shake

In a Blender Combine:

+ FLUID

> 1 Cup / 8ozs of water, Add 3-4 cubes of ice. (If using frozen fruit skip this step)

+ FAT

> 1 tablespoon of flaxseed oil, grape seed oil or an avocado

+ PROTIEN

> Clean Protein Powder. (Whey, Pea or a combo Pea and Rice)

+ FIBER

> This step can be optional if you have a sensitive stomach

+ FRUIT

> 1 Cup of fruit, (frozen fruit makes the shake thicker) Choose berries, apple, pineapple, kiwi and or a ½ of a banana

+ VEGGIES

> 2 Cups of veggies: spinach, kale, celery, cucumber, parsley, beets or carrot etc.

+ SPICE

> Use a squeeze of lemon or lime, grated ginger, vanilla extract, cinnamon, or mint etc.

+ BLEND

> Use a high performance Blender to mix all the ingredients and enjoy!

A SAMPLE MENU FOR THE WEEK

MONDAY

Breakfast: The Ultimate Protein Smoothie

Mid Morning Snack: Kale Chips

Lunch: Roasted Root Veggies with Lemon Dill Dressing

Mid Afternoon: The Ultimate Protein Smoothie

Dinner: Dr. Pia's Super Salad

TUESDAY

Breakfast: The Ultimate Protein Smoothie

Mid Morning Snack: A piece of approved fruit

Lunch: Asian Slaw with Ginger Lime Dressing

Mid Afternoon: The Ultimate Protein Smoothie

Dinner: Grilled Veggies with Mashed Avocado

WEDNESDAY

Breakfast: The Ultimate Protein Smoothie

Mid Morning: Approved Fruit

Lunch: Asian Zucchini Zoodle Salad

Mid Afternoon: The Ultimate Protein Smoothie

Dinner: Loaded Lentil and Carrot Soup

THURSDAY

Breakfast: The Ultimate Protein Smoothie

Mid Morning Snack: kale Chips

Lunch: Raw kale salad with Root Veggies with curry vinaigrette

Mid Afternoon: The Ultimate Protein Smoothie

Dinner: Chicken Sir Fry (Day 11-21)

FRIDAY

Breakfast: The Ultimate Protein Smoothie

Mid Morning: Approved Fruit

Lunch: Veggie Wraps

Mid Afternoon: The Ultimate Protein Smoothie

Dinner: Baked Sea Bass with Veggies (11-21)

SATURDAY

Breakfast: The Ultimate Protein Smoothie

Mid Morning: Cauliflower Hummus

Lunch: Grilled sweet potato Fries with Cruciferous Veggies

Mid Afternoon: The Ultimate Protein Smoothie

Dinner: Cajun Salmon with Lemon Pepper Asparagus (Day 11-21)

SUNDAY

Breakfast: The Ultimate Protein Smoothie

Mid Morning Snack: kale Chips

Lunch: Spicy Chicken Soup with Veggies (Day 11-21)

Mid Afternoon: The Ultimate Protein Smoothie

Dinner: A Buddha Bowl

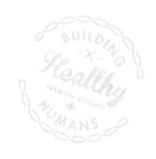

MAINTAINING GOOD HEALTH POST P21

Congratulations! You have cleansed your liver, kidneys, lungs, blood, skin and bowels and your body loves you for it! This is probably the best you have felt in a long time!

You are now ready for the next step! Now you can apply what you have learned and move forward to a healthier attitude toward food for a lifetime. You have learned that good clean organic foods are like medicine for the body and they have the power to heal from the inside out.

This is where we suggest you start taking the BHH pre-natal packs for added pre-conception nutrients.

If you have been struggling with Hormonal health problems and have been having trouble conceiving we suggest you continue to follow days 11-21 of the P21program for a healthier more nutritious way of eating, living and being. We know you are on the road to a beautiful and balanced pregnancy and a happy healthy baby.

The key to your new normal eating plan is the re-introduction of certain foods. You should continue to follow the 11-21 day meal plan and slowly add one food group at a time. It is highly possible that some of the foods you were eating prior to P21 program were not the best for you. It is also possible that you had a food sensitivity or intolerance that you didn't know about.

We have laid out a plan below that is the best way we have found to introduce certain foods groups back into your diet. You will want to pay close attention to how you feel and if you notice any changes.

UNDERSTANDING FOOD SENSITIVITIES. A FOOD RE-INTRODUCTION PLAN

We begin by adding one food group per week.

Week One: Grain:

Add ½ a cup of brown rice a day to your plan.

Week Two: Nuts and Seeds

Add a small handful of toasted or raw almonds and or sunflower or pumpkin seeds a day to your plan.

Week Three: Pulses and Legumes

Add beans and peas to your food options.

Week Four: Organic non-cow Dairy.

Add one oz. of goat cheese to your food options per day.

Week Five: Organic Free Range Eggs.

Eggs provide an important and easy to digest source of protein, iron and B vitamins.

We recommend that you DO NOT add back known inflammatory and highly processed foods. We also suggest that you continue to eliminate Wheat, Cow Dairy, Soy, Corn and Alcohol until after you have had your baby. Even then do so using a slow process of introduction. Pay close attention to any changes and if you are breast-feeding pay close attention to any changes in baby.

Most of us understand an allergic reaction to certain foods.

There are two types of inflammatory "reactions" that apply to most people. The first one (IgE) is immediate and the second one (IgG) is delayed.

An immediate response to a food you are allergic to might present itself through symptoms such as sneezing, runny nose, red eyes, increased heart rate, hives, nausea, or migraines.

The solution to this problem is to simply avoid eating these foods!

The other type of response is food intolerance, which is more insidious and difficult to identify. It is "the delayed reaction" type of food intolerance.

This IgG reaction can take hours, even days to express itself. For example, you eat wheat on Monday and all that day, all day Tuesday and even part of Wednesday you feel fine. Then, on Wednesday evening your migraines are back, or your joints are on fire, or your irritable bowel rears its ugly head. You wouldn't normally make the connection between the food you are eating (or in this example 'ate') and your symptoms, but there seems to be a strong connection between these delayed food allergies and many chronic health concerns.

As if that is not enough, here is another rub. **You may actually be addicted to or craving the very foods to which you are intolerant.**

They give you kind of an adrenaline rush! You feel almost euphoric or high after eating them only to crash afterwards, feeling drained and miserable.

Research tells us what are the most common food sensitivities and allergens, however we all have a unique blueprint and therefore what is OK for some is not OK for others. Wheat or Soy would be a good example of how we differ.

It is helpful to keep a food experience log and notice how certain foods make you feel after you have introduced them. During the introduction period you should weigh each day at the same time. If you have gained 2-3 pounds seemingly overnight it is usually a sign that the food you ingested has caused low-grade inflammation in the body. The body will hold onto water to protect vital organs and it will show up as weight fluid gain.

The most common food allergies or intolerance are: peanuts, shellfish, milk, eggs, soy and wheat and other gluten-containing grains. You can also experience food intolerances to certain additives in food like MSG or derivatives of sugars like Aspartame.

Healthy For A Lifetime

Maintaining your weight and staying healthy and looking good is a lifelong commitment and sometimes the journey is not always easy. The key is to be mindful and realize that it's the small choices we make every day that count. Beating your self up does not work, but getting back on track does.

Here are some tips to help you with your life long goal of a healthy life:

- Prepare for social gatherings and travel. Planning ahead is key.
- It's Ok to give into cravings once a while. Just make it a treat and then get back on track. The idea is to re-think your relationship with food.
- Aim to stick to foods that are found in to nature. Keep refined and processed foods out of the house so you won't be tempted.
- Keep alcohol and coffee to a minimum, as they can easily become habit-forming
- Watch portion size and eat slowly.
- Read labels. Or better yet don't eat package or processed food. Your well-being depends on it. Ever look at what's in a loaf of bread?
- Fill in any nutritional gaps with our Pre-Natal or Dr. Pia's Top 5. We recommend a good multivitamin, an Omega 3 Fatty

Acid, Vitamin D, Trace Mineral B12 and a Probiotic. Add B12 if you follow a vegetarian or vegan diet

We Suggest You Continue your Shakes for Optimal Health

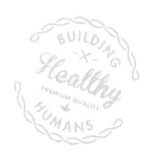

YOUR EXPERIENCE JOURNAL

Day One: Blast Off! Here we go!

What did you eat and drink today?

Breakfast: _____

_____

Lunch: _____

_____

Dinner: _____

_____

Other: _____

_____

How do you feel? _____

_____

Did you exercise? How long? _____

_____

Are you experiencing any physical or emotional effects?_____

_____

Day Two: Ouch! I would kill for a coffee right now.

What did you eat and drink today?

Breakfast: _____

_____

Lunch: _____

_____

Dinner: _____

_____

Other: _____

_____

How do you feel? _____

_____

Did you exercise? How long? _____

_____

Are you experiencing any physical or emotional effects?_____

_____

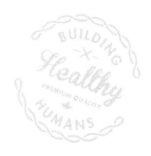

Day Three: A little pooped today!

What did you eat and drink today?

Breakfast: _____

_____

Lunch: _____

_____

Dinner: _____

_____

Other: _____

_____

How do you feel? _____

_____

Did you exercise? How long? _____

_____

Are you experiencing any physical or emotional effects?_____

_____

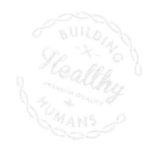

Day Four: Oh! It has been a long three days, but I am kicking those toxins to the curb.

What did you eat and drink today?

Breakfast: _____

_____

Lunch: _____

_____

Dinner: _____

_____

Other: _____

_____

How do you feel? _____

_____

Did you exercise? How long? _____

_____

Are you experiencing any physical or emotional effects?_____

_____

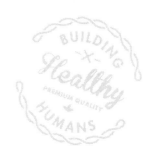

Day Five: Finally starting to feel lighter and brighter.

What did you eat and drink today?

Breakfast: _____

_____

Lunch: _____

_____

Dinner: _____

_____

Other: _____

_____

How do you feel? _____

_____

Did you exercise? How long? _____

_____

Are you experiencing any physical or emotional effects?_____

_____

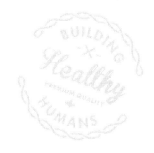

Day Six: Loving those dark leafy greens

What did you eat and drink today?

Breakfast: _____

_____

Lunch: _____

_____

Dinner: _____

_____

Other: _____

_____

How do you feel? _____

_____

Did you exercise? How long? _____

_____

Are you experiencing any physical or emotional effects?_____

_____

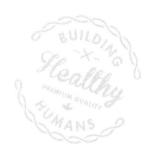

Day Seven: Whew! I made it. One week down and getting my body ready to build a healthy human.

What did you eat and drink today?

Breakfast: _____

_____

Lunch: _____

_____

Dinner: _____

_____

Other: _____

_____

How do you feel? _____

_____

Did you exercise? How long? _____

_____

Are you experiencing any physical or emotional effects?_____

_____

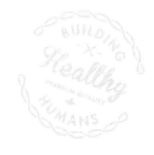

Day Eight: On a roll! Bring it on!

What did you eat and drink today?

Breakfast: _____

_____

Lunch: _____

_____

Dinner: _____

_____

Other: _____

_____

How do you feel? _____

_____

Did you exercise? How long? _____

_____

Are you experiencing any physical or emotional effects?_____

_____

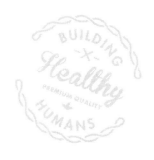

Day Nine: This is the most veggies I have eaten in my life!

What did you eat and drink today?

Breakfast: _____

_____

Lunch: _____

_____

Dinner: _____

_____

Other: _____

_____

How do you feel? _____

_____

Did you exercise? How long? _____

_____

Are you experiencing any physical or emotional effects?_____

_____

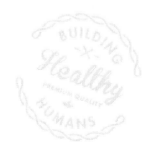

Day Ten: Dreaming of protein

What did you eat and drink today?

Breakfast: _____

_____

Lunch: _____

_____

Dinner: _____

_____

Other: _____

_____

How do you feel? _____

_____

Did you exercise? How long? _____

_____

Are you experiencing any physical or emotional effects?_____

_____

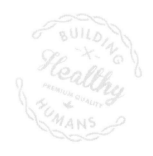

Day Eleven: Ahhh! Three ounces of fish or chicken, or an egg!

What did you eat and drink today?

Breakfast: _____

_____

Lunch: _____

_____

Dinner: _____

_____

Other: _____

_____

How do you feel? _____

_____

Did you exercise? How long? _____

_____

Are you experiencing any physical or emotional effects?_____

_____

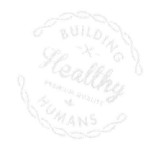

Day Twelve: Did the protein. No big deal. Bring on the fruit and veggies

What did you eat and drink today?

Breakfast: _____

_____

Lunch: _____

_____

Dinner: _____

_____

Other: _____

_____

How do you feel? _____

_____

Did you exercise? How long? _____

_____

Are you experiencing any physical or emotional effects?_____

_____

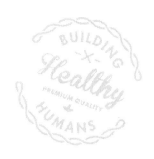

Day Thirteen: Getting the hang of this and I can feel my genes thanking me.

What did you eat and drink today?

Breakfast: _____

_____

Lunch: _____

_____

Dinner: _____

_____

Other: _____

_____

How do you feel? _____

_____

Did you exercise? How long? _____

_____

Are you experiencing any physical or emotional effects?_____

_____

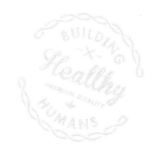

Day Fourteen: Dinner out with my friends and I notice how much mindless eating they are doing!

What did you eat and drink today?

Breakfast: _____

_____

Lunch: _____

_____

Dinner: _____

_____

Other: _____

_____

How do you feel? _____

_____

Did you exercise? How long? _____

_____

Are you experiencing any physical or emotional effects?_____

_____

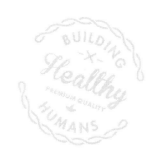

Day Fifteen: Random strangers stop me and tell me how good my skin looks!

What did you eat and drink today?

Breakfast: _____

_____

Lunch: _____

_____

Dinner: _____

_____

Other: _____

_____

How do you feel? _____

_____

Did you exercise? How long? _____

_____

Are you experiencing any physical or emotional effects?_____

_____

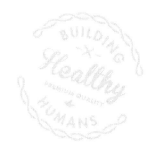

Day Sixteen: I noticed that I don't have any aches or pains in my joints.

What did you eat and drink today?

Breakfast: _____

_____

Lunch: _____

_____

Dinner: _____

_____

Other: _____

_____

How do you feel? _____

_____

Did you exercise? How long? _____

_____

Are you experiencing any physical or emotional effects?_____

_____

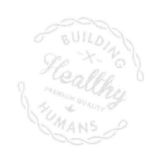

Day Seventeen: My clothes are loose and it's time to go shopping!

What did you eat and drink today?

Breakfast: _____

_____

Lunch: _____

_____

Dinner: _____

_____

Other: _____

_____

How do you feel? _____

_____

Did you exercise? How long? _____

_____

Are you experiencing any physical or emotional effects?_____

_____

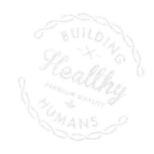

Day Eighteen: I have increased energy, and my allergies are gone.

What did you eat and drink today?

Breakfast: _____

_____

Lunch: _____

_____

Dinner: _____

_____

Other: _____

_____

How do you feel? _____

_____

Did you exercise? How long? _____

_____

Are you experiencing any physical or emotional effects?_____

_____

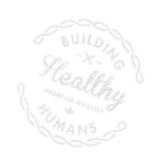

Day Nineteen: I could get used to this!

What did you eat and drink today?

Breakfast: _____

_____

Lunch: _____

_____

Dinner: _____

_____

Other: _____

_____

How do you feel? _____

_____

Did you exercise? How long? _____

_____

Are you experiencing any physical or emotional effects?_____

_____

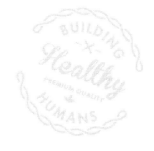

Day Twenty: I feel great! People at work are noticing my vitality and ask, "What have you been doing?"

What did you eat and drink today?

Breakfast: _____

_____

Lunch: _____

_____

Dinner: _____

_____

Other: _____

_____

How do you feel? _____

_____

Did you exercise? How long? _____

_____

Are you experiencing any physical or emotional effects?_____

_____

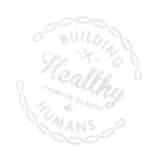

Day Twenty-One: I made it! Now I know that food is medicine and I feel great! I am telling everyone I know that they should do this if they want to build a healthy human.

What did you eat and drink today?

Breakfast: _____

_____

Lunch: _____

_____

Dinner: _____

_____

Other: _____

_____

How do you feel? _____

_____

Did you exercise? How long? _____

_____

Are you experiencing any physical or emotional effects?_____

_____

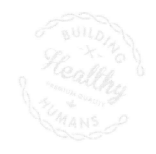

145

Day Twenty-Two: Formed some great new habits and I am ready to continue eating clean!

What did you eat and drink today?

Breakfast: _____

_____

Lunch: _____

_____

Dinner: _____

_____

Other: _____

_____

How do you feel? _____

_____

Did you exercise? How long? _____

_____

Are you experiencing any physical or emotional effects?_____

_____

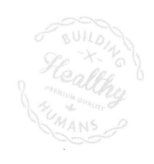

RECIPES

Kale Chips

- 1 bunch kale, stems removed, torn into bite-size pieces
- 1 tablespoon olive oil
- 1 teaspoon sea salt

Preheat oven to 350 F. With your fingers, carefully remove the kale leaves from the thick stems and tear into bite-size pieces. Drizzle kale with olive oil and massage oil into the kale. Spread out evenly on cookie sheet and sprinkle with sea salt. Place in the oven for 10 minutes or until crispy. **Serves 2.**

Roasted Root Veggies with Lemon Dill Sauce

- Bunch of red and gold beets, cut into quarters
- 2 carrots cut in half and then cut length wise
- One medium turnip cut into quarters

Preheat the oven to 400 degrees. Toss veggies in olive oil, and set onto a lines roasting pan. Sprinkle on seas salt and celery seeds. Cook till tender. **Makes 2 servings.**

Lemon Dill Dressing

- 3 tablespoons fresh lemon juice
- 1 teaspoon Dijon mustard (no sugar)
- ½ teaspoon dill weed
- ¼ teaspoon hot pepper sauce

In a small bowl, whisk together all ingredients thoroughly. **Makes 1 serving.**

Dr. Pia's Super Salad

- 2 medium carrots shredded
- 1 red beet shredded
- 3 handfuls of organic mixed green leaves
- Chopped cilantro, parsley and mint leaves
- A large avocado peeled and cubed

- 2 cups of bite size pieces of steamed Broccoli
- 4 Roasted Brussels sprouts chopped
- 4 spring onions finely chopped
- Sea salt
- 1 tablespoon plus 2 teaspoons fresh ginger, minced

Add all ingredients into a large bowl and toss with your favorite dressing. **Serves 2**

Asian Slaw With Warm Ginger Lime Dressing

- 6 cups thinly sliced cabbage, any variety
- 2 medium carrots, peeled and cut into very thin matchsticks
- 1 apple, peeled and cut into thin matchsticks
- ½ teaspoon sea salt
- 3 tablespoons apple cider vinegar
- 2 tablespoons plus 1-teaspoon fresh lime juice

- 2 tablespoons water
- 2 tablespoons olive oil
- 1 large red onion, thinly sliced
- Sea salt
- 1 tablespoon plus 2 teaspoons fresh ginger, minced
- ½ cup (packed) fresh cilantro, stems removed, divided

In a large bowl, combine cabbage, carrots, and apple. Sprinkle with salt to taste. In a small bowl, whisk together vinegar, lime juice, 2 tablespoons water. In a skillet, heat oil over medium heat. Add onion and salt and cook 6-8 minutes until onion is browned. Add vinegar mixture and ginger, and then cook for another 30 seconds. Remove from heat. Add onion mixture to cabbage mixture. Toss until well combined and cabbage begins to wilt. Add half of the cilantro leaves and toss to combine. Let this stand for about 5 minutes, then serve, garnished with remaining cilantro. **Serves 6.**

Grilled Veggies with Avocado Mash

- Two zucchini cut in half then lengthwise.
- handful of asparagus washed and trimmed
- One Red Peeper
- One Portobello Mushroom
- 6 partial steamed Brussels sprouts

Prepare the grill. Drizzle on your favorite good for you oil, add some spice and sprinkle with sea salt. Grill till tender and serve with Avocado Mash. **Makes 2 servings.**

Chicken Stir-Fry

For the marinade: ¼ cup coconut milk 3 tablespoons balsamic vinegar 1 tablespoon olive oil 2 tablespoons fresh ginger, minced 3 cloves garlic, chopped Salt and pepper

- 2 pounds chicken, cut into strips
- 3 tablespoons coconut oil, divided
- 3 cups broccoli, chopped
- 1 cup mushrooms, chopped 3 celery stalks, chopped 1 cup snap peas
- 2 teaspoons sesame oil ½ cup water chestnuts
- 3 scallions, chopped
- Sea salt and pepper

In a small bowl, mix all marinade ingredients and transfer to shallow at dish. Add the chicken and marinate for 15-30 minutes. In a large skillet, heat 1 tablespoon coconut oil over medium heat. Cook the broccoli for 3-4 minutes, then remove from pan and set aside. Add remaining coconut oil and stir-fry the mushrooms, celery, and snap peas for 2-3 minutes. Remove and set aside. Remove chicken from marinade and add to the skillet along with sesame oil. Cook the chicken over medium heat until completely white, about 5-7 minutes. Add water chestnuts and scallions, and mix well. Season lightly with sea salt and pepper. Serve immediately. Serves 4.

Raw Kale Salad With Root Vegetables

- 2 (12-ounce) bunches kale, stems removed, leaves cut into thin strips
- 2 tablespoons olive oil or nut oil
- 1 tablespoon apple cider vinegar
- 1 teaspoon sea salt
- 1 medium turnip, peeled, grated
- ½ medium rutabaga, peeled, grated
- 1 medium beet (red or golden), peeled, grated
- 1 medium carrot, grated
- 2 green onions cut thin on diagonal
- 2 tablespoons fresh lemon juice
- 1 tablespoon fresh lemon zest
- 1 tablespoon olive oil
- 1 tablespoon balsamic vinegar
- 1 teaspoon whole-leaf stevia powder
- Sea salt and ground pepper (optional)

Place kale in a large bowl and add in olive oil, vinegar, and sea salt. Gently massage mixture into kale about 2-3 minutes by hand or until kale starts to wilt. Let rest 30 minutes. Stir turnip, rutabaga, beet, carrot, and green onions into kale mixture. In a Bowl whisk all of the dressing ingredients. Season with salt and pepper if desired.

Add dressing to kale salad and toss thoroughly. Garnish with pecans if desired. **Serves 6.**

Loaded Carrot and Lentil Soup

- 1 ¼ cups red lentils
- 3 tablespoons of ghee
- 1 red onion, chopped
- 1 clove garlic, chopped
- 2 tablespoons sun-dried tomato purée
- 1 pound carrots, grated
- 3 quarts of organic vegetable stock
- Fresh cilantro chopped

Rinse and drains the lentils, then set aside. Heat the butter with the onion and garlic, cooking for 4-5 minutes. Add the sun-dried tomato purée and cook for 1 minute. Add carrots, lentils, and stock and bring to a boil. Cook at a rapid simmer for 40 minutes or until the lentils are soft. Spoon the soup, in batches, into a food processor, or blender and process until smooth. Return the soup to a clean pan and cook over a low heat for a few minutes or until heated through. Serve in bowls topped with fresh cilantro. **Serves 4.**

Cauliflower Hummus

- 1 head of Cauliflower cut into florets and steamed
- ½ cup of Tahini
- 1 Clove of garlic peeled
- Juice of 2 lemons
- Seal salt
- 1 teaspoon of Cumin
- ½ cup of olive oil

Add all ingredients to a food processer or Vitamix and blend till the mixture is the consistency of hummus. Adjust liquid as needed.

Veggie Wraps

- Washed and stems removed of Collard Greens
- Avocado mashed
- Red onion minced
- Cucumber thinly sliced
- Carrot grated
- Radish grated
- Cauliflower hummus. See the recipe above.

Layer the ingredients on the Collard green leave and fold the top and the bottom inwards and lightly roll into a wrap. This is a great way to include left overs for a healthy lunch.

Cajun Salmon

- Olive oil or coconut oil
- 2 medium-sized pieces of salmon
- 2 teaspoons ground cumin
- 2 teaspoons ground coriander
- 1 clove garlic, minced
- 1 teaspoon paprika
- ½ teaspoon cayenne pepper
- ½ teaspoon dried thyme
- 2 teaspoons oregano
- Sea salt and ground pepper

In a medium sauté pan, heat oil at medium-high heat. In a small bowl, combine the spices. Turn the salmon in the spices, covering all sides. Place the salmon filets (skin side under) in pan. Cook for 3-5 minutes before turning over. Cook another 3-4 minutes or until done. **Serves 2.**

Lemon Pepper Asparagus

- 2 tablespoons coconut oil
- 3 pounds fresh asparagus, chopped,
- 2 cloves garlic, chopped
- ¼ cup fresh lemon juice
- Zest from lemon
- Salt and pepper

In a large skillet, heat oil over high heat. Stir-fry asparagus and garlic until crisp yet tender. Reduce heat to medium. Add lemon juice, zest, salt, and pepper. Cover and let steam for 2-3 minutes. You may steam up to 10 minutes to yield a soft, delicate avor. **Serves 4.**

Grilled Sweet Potatoes Fries with Cruciferous Veggies

- 1 Sweet potato cut into thick finger fries
- An assortment of Lightly steamed Broccoli, Cauliflower, and Brussels sprouts

Toss all the veggies in a marinade of olive oil, sea salt lemon and celery seed. Heat grill and cook till tender serve with a Dijon Mustard sauce.

Spicy Chicken Soup with Veggies

- 1 whole chicken
- 1 Quart of low sodium organic broth and 2 Quarts of water
- 2 cloves garlic, crushed
- 2 onions roughly chopped
- 2 Celery stalks roughly chopped
- 2 medium carrots chopped into 3 chunks
- 2 sprigs of Thyme and 6 parsley stems
- 1 small knob of ginger sliced

- 1 tsp of cumin and I tsp of all spice
- Sprinkle of re chili flakes
- Sea salt and pepper

Place Chicken in a large stock pot and add the above ingredients. Bring to boil and simmer for one hour. Chicken should pull away from bones. Remove Chicken and set aside to cool. Strain the broth thru a fine mesh sieve and set aside. Discard the veggies. When chicken has cooled shred into piece and set aside.

- 2 Tablespoons of Coconut oil
- 4 button mushrooms
- 1 small onions sliced
- 1 Celery stalk diced
- 1 medium carrot sliced
- Fresh Parsley chopped for garnish and or Sliced Avocado
- 1 bunch of spinach roughly chopped (You can use Kale or Cabbage)
- Sea salt and pepper

Melt oil in a stockpot, add mushrooms and cook 3 mins, then add diced onion, carrots, celery and cook until veggies are softened. Add reserved chicken, and chicken stock and bring to the boil. Add kale, spinach or cabbage and cook until wilted. Remove from heat add parsley add sliced Avocado if you like and serve hot

Asian Zucchini Zoodle Salad

- 3-4 Zucchinis
- 1 ½ cups of shredded red cabbage
- 1 Carrot grated
- 1 teaspoon sea salt
- ½ red bell pepper thinly sliced
- 12 Green opinions thinly sliced
- ½ a bunch of Cilantro leaves chopped
- Rice Vinegar
- Olive oil
- Sesame oil
- 1 teaspoon of minced garlic
- pinch of re chili flakes

Make the zucchini noodles using a spiralizer or sclizer. Sprinkle with salt salt and drain for 30 minutes. Toss with all other ingredients in a large Medium bowl and serve.

Baked Sea Bass With Vegetables

- 1 tablespoon olive oil or coconut oil
- 4 sea bass lfillets
- 2 cloves garlic, chopped
- 1 onion, sliced
- 4 cups spinach leaves
- 4 carrots chopped into 3 chunks

- ⅛ cup green onions, chopped
- 15 stems of asparagus
- 1 zucchini, sliced
- 1 sweet potato, cooked, sliced in ¼ inch slices
- 1 teaspoon dried dill weed
- Sea salt and pepper

Preheat oven to 350 F. Massage oil into the fish, then place l in baking dish. Lay all remaining ingredients except dill weed, salt, and pepper over fish. Sprinkle with dill weed and salt and pepper to taste. Cover dish with parchment paper and bake for approximately 30 minutes or until vegetables are soft and fish flake easily. **Serves 4.**

A Buddha Bowl

- 3 handfuls of raw organic greens (Kale, Micro Greens and Arugula)
- Roasted Spring Onions
- 2 Cups of roasted Veggies chopped in bite size pieces (Sweet potatoes, beets, Brussels sprouts etc.

- ½ cup of raw shredded purple cabbage
- ½ cup of cooked cumin spiced lentils
- ½ Avocado
- 2 hard-boiled eggs chopped in half

155

- ¼ teaspoon cayenne pepper
- ½ cup of cilantro chopped
- Lemon Juice
- Sea salt and ground pepper

In a large unique bowl, layer in the raw greens, then around the edges in a clockwise direction add roasted veggies, lentils, cabbage, and spring onions. Layer on the top the chopped hard-boiled eggs. Mix the Avocado, lemon cilantro and spices and drizzle on top of your Buddha Bowl. **Serves 2.**

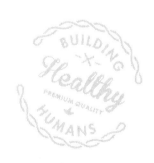

DOCTOR PIA'S PLANT BASED PALEO DIET

- Focus on the glycemic load of your diet.

- Focus on more protein and fats. Nuts (not peanuts), seeds (flax, chia, hemp, sesame, pumpkin), coconut, avocados, sardines, olive oil.

- Eat the right fats. Stay away from most vegetable oils such as canola, sunflower, corn, and especially soybean oil, which now comprises about 10 percent of our calories.

- Focus instead on omega 3 fats, nuts, coconut, and avocados and yes, even saturated fat from grass fed or sustainably raised animals.

- Eat mostly plants – lots of low glycemic vegetables and fruits. This should be 75 percent of your diet and your plate. I usually make 2 to 3 vegetable dishes per meal. Add to a bowl of leafy greens for added nutrients

- Focus on nuts and seeds. They are full of protein, minerals, and good fats and they lower the risk of heart disease and diabetes.

- Avoid dairy – it is for growing calves into cows, not for humans. Try goat or sheep products, only as a treat and always organic.

- Avoid gluten –if you are not gluten sensitive, then consider it an occasional treat and look for sprouted sources.

- Eat gluten-free whole grains sparingly – Quinoa, buckwheat etc as they still raise blood sugar and can trigger autoimmunity.

- Eat beans sparingly – lentils are best. Stay away from big starchy beans.

- Eat organic and wild sources of meat, fish or fowl. Vegetables should take center stage and meat/ fish or fowl should be a side dish.

- Think of sugar as an occasional treat – Honey, palm sugar etc. Sugar free would be best and it is very addictive and hard for most to have as a treat.

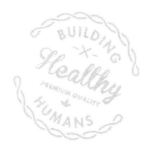

ULTIMATE PROTEIN SHAKE RECIPES

How to make the base for the Ultimate Protein Shake.

In a Blender Combine:

+ FLUID

1 Cup/8ozs. of water, unsweetened coconut or hemp milk.

Add 3-4 cubes of ice or freeze the milk. (If using frozen fruit skip this step).

+ FAT

1 tablespoon of Flaxseed oil, grape seed oil or an avocado.

+ PROTIEN

Whey Protein Powder, Pea Protein or SP Complete Handful of nuts.

+ FIBER

This step can be optional if you have a sensitive stomach.

+ FRUIT

1 Cup of Fruit, (Frozen Fruit makes the shake thicker) Choose Berries, Apple, Pineapple, Orange, Kiwi and or a ½ of a Banana.

+ VEGGIES

2 Cups of veggies: Spinach, Kale, Celery, Cucumber, Parsley, or Carrot etc.

+ SPICE

Use Lemon, Lime, Ginger, Vanilla Extract, cinnamon, or Mint etc.

Some Sample combinations

- Protein Powder
- Water
- Frozen Berries
- ½ of a Banana
- Flax seed oil
- Spinach

- Protein Powder
- Water
- Avocado
- ½ of a Banana
- Spinach or Kale
- Walnuts
- Ginger

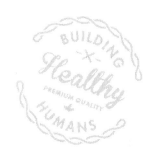

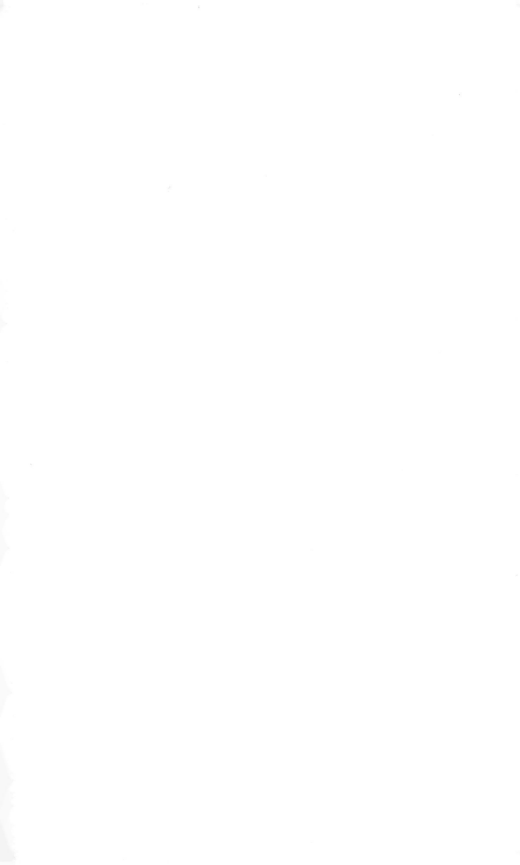

Made in the USA
San Bernardino, CA
24 September 2017